KU-865-588

Teaching Physical Skills for the Childbearing Year

Eileen Brayshaw MCSP, SRP, FETC

Superintendent Physiotherapist, St James's University Hospital, Leeds

&

Pauline Wright MCSP, SRP, FETC

Former Superintendent Physiotherapist, South Birmingham Womens' Health Unit,

MEDICAL LIBRARY
WATFORD POSTGRADUATE
MEDICAL CENTRE
WATFORD GENERAL HOSPITAL
VICARAGE ROAD
WATFORD WD1 8HB

Books for Midwives Press

Books for Midwives Press is a joint publishing venture between
The Royal College of Midwives and Haigh & Hochland Publications Ltd

©1994 Eileen Brayshaw and Pauline Wright

First Edition

All rights reserved. No part of this book may be reproduced in any form or by any electronic or mechanical means, including information storage and retrieval systems, without permission in writing from the publisher, except by a reviewer who may quote brief passages in a review.

ISBN 1-898507-02-3

British Library Cataloguing in Publication Data
A catalogue record for this book is available from the British Library

Anatomical drawings by the Medical Art Department, The Royal Marsden Hospital, London

Printed in the UK by RAP Ltd

Published by Books for Midwives Press, 174A Ashley Road, Hale, Cheshire, England WA15 9SF

Contents

Preface

We have written this book in response to requests from midwives, health visitors and others who are expected to teach physical preparation for childbirth without the help of an obstetric physiotherapist. Many of these parenthood educators lack the expertise and background knowledge needed to teach physical skills with confidence. They should understand the rationale for including these skills in the preparation for parenthood, before attempting to teach them. We have therefore incorporated a basic description of the relevant physiology, and of the anatomy and functions of those muscles especially involved during the childbearing year.

Having gained the above knowledge the reader can then move on to the subsequent chapters to learn and practise performing the basic exercises, relaxation and coping strategies. A later chapter describes how to teach these physical skills to individuals and small groups. The prospective teacher should then evaluate her personal performance before progressing to instructing larger groups.

We have intentionally repeated the exercises in both the ante and postnatal chapters so that each chapter can stand independently. Chapter 9 embraces all the information relating to the exercises in Chapters 3 and 8 in a comprehensive package for easy referral. This chapter also includes additional antenatal and stretching exercises.

Also included in this first comprehensive illustrated guide for those teaching essential physical skills in preparation for parenthood, are chapters on programme-planning, transcutaneous electrical nerve stimulation (TENS), aquanatal exercises and exercises to music. We hope that the information provided is easy to assimilate and will enable teachers to approach their groups with increased confidence.

We wish to thank Georgina Evans, Barbara LeRoy, Jeanne McIntosh and Betty Sweet for their invaluable help and support, Sue Barton for her initial exercise illustrations and Henry, Des and Jo for their continued encouragement and forbearance.

History of Physical Preparation for Childbirth

As far back as 1912 Minnie Randell, head of St. Thomas's school of physiotherapy, and also a midwife, was asked by Dr. Fairbairn, an obstetrician, to teach postnatal exercises in order to aid physical recovery and to encourage rest and relaxation.

A physical routine was then established antenatally to promote physical health and help prevent problems. Minnie Randell was further influenced by Dr. Kathleen Vaughan who encouraged the teaching of stretching exercises to increase mobility of the pelvic joints and lumbar spine. Positions of comfort were also introduced to facilitate labour.

From the 1930s, the pioneer Grantly Dick-Read, voiced his theory of the fear-tension-pain cycle in labour. He included very little general exercise in his training programme, but emphasis was placed on women learning to relax and breathe deeply through contractions.

Minnie Randell followed this regime and in partnership with Margaret Morris, a ballet dancer, encouraged women to rehearse for the performance of labour. Helen Heardman, another teacher of physiotherapy, based her teaching on ideas from both St. Thomas's and from Grantly Dick-Read. In the 1940s she offered courses for labour and parenthood which included education, relaxation and breathing.

In the 1950s, psychoprophylaxis became fashionable. This was a new trend which came to Britain from Russia via Paris. A very rigid training was taught and included controlled patterns (levels) of breathing. It was only a preparation for labour; postnatal rehabilitation was not included as part of the course.

In common with other forms of education, there has been a move from authoritarian didactic teaching to "a client led" approach. Both women and partners now attend psychophysical preparation classes and express their physical and emotional needs for inclusion in the programme. Relaxation, breathing and exercises are always requested. This book concentrates on these.

Over the years there have been discussions between the Royal College of Midwives, the Health Visitors Association and the Chartered Society of Physiotherapy about each members' roles in Psychophysical Preparation, and the latest Tripartite Agreement is as follows:

Statement by the Royal College of Midwives, the Health Visitors Association and the Chartered Society of Physiotherapy on:

WORKING TOGETHER IN PSYCHOPHYSICAL PREPARATION FOR CHILDBIRTH

1. Midwives, health visitors and obstetric physiotherapists all have important specialist contributions to make in the preparation for childbirth and parenthood. This contact with parents also provides a valuable opportunity for more general health promotion, health education and preventative medicine. In the delivery of such a service in any locality, it is important that the professional team demonstrates a flexible approach and takes account of the views and needs of all parents.

2. The role of the midwife is that of the practitioner of normal midwifery, caring for the woman within the hospital and community throughout the continuum of pregnancy, childbirth and the puerperium. She has an important contribution to make in health education, counselling and support. In this context her aim is to facilitate the realisation of women's needs, discuss expectations and air anxieties. She has the responsibility of monitoring the woman's physical, psychological and social wellbeing and is in a unique position to be able to correlate parent education with midwifery care.

3. The role of the health visitor in this field is to offer advice to the parents-to-be on the many health, psychological and social implications of becoming parents and the development of the child. She is in a very special position in the family scene to inform them of the services available and to encourage them to use them. The health visitor should always have a participatory role within the team to provide continuity of care to the family.

4. The role of the obstetric physiotherapist is to promote health during the childbearing period and to help the woman adjust advantageously to the physical and psychological changes of pregnancy and the postnatal period so that the stresses of childbearing are minimised. Antenatally and postnatally she advises on physical activity associated with both work and leisure and is a specialist in selecting and teaching appropriate exercises to gain and/or maintain fitness including pelvic-floor education. Where necessary she gives specialised treatment

e.g. therapeutic ultrasound postnatally to alleviate discomfort. She also assesses and treats musculo-skeletal problems such as backache and pelvic-floor muscle weakness. In addition she is a skilled teacher of effective relaxation, breathing awareness and positioning and thus helps the woman to prepare for labour.

5.   In order for the services of the team to be of maximum benefit to parents there should be a close liaison between its members. Liaison, planning and shared learning sessions help to ensure that techniques and advice are consistent, up-to-date, relate to current practice and meet the needs of the parents. This is particularly important when there is no available member of one of the specialist professions. Where this is the case, advice should be sought from the relevant professional body. To enhance continuity of care, new members of the team must always have a period of inter-disciplinary induction. The midwife, health visitor and obstetric physiotherapist should be in regular contact and operate an effective referral system.

6.   The aims of parenthood education are summarised as follows:
   • To enable parents to develop a confident and relaxed approach to pregnancy, childbirth and parenthood.
   • To enable parents to be aware of the choices in care based on accurate and up-to-date information.
   • To provide continuity of high quality care, as previously defined to parents, by means of team collaboration and cooperation between professionals including specialised treatments where needed.
   • To ensure that appropriate, consistent and clear advice is given with full cognisance of safety factors.
   • To promote health and preventative medicine.

Frequently new methods of education in parenthood are introduced e.g. aquanatal and fitness classes. In such instances it is necessary for guidance to be sought from the local obstetric physiotherapist or alternatively from the Chartered Society of Physiotherapy, and further training may be required.

January 1994

CHAPTER 1

Pelvic

Anatomy

This chapter contains the anatomy relevant as background knowledge for those teaching physical skills in preparation for parenthood.

THE PELVIS

The pelvis is the bony ring at the base of the trunk. It is made up of four bones - the **coccyx**, **sacrum** and two large **innominate** or **hip bones**. Three parts make up each innominate bone - the **ilium**, **ischium** and **pubis**. The sacrum, a wedge-shaped bone made up of five rudimentary **sacral vertebrae**, joins the two iliac bones at the part-synovial, part-fibrous **sacroiliac joints**. The joint joining the two pubic bones anteriorly is the cartilaginous **symphysis pubis** and the coccyx (usually composed of four rudimentary coccygeal vertebrae) is attached to the sacrum at the **sacrococcygeal joint.** As well as these joints linking the bones of the pelvis together, the rest of the spine is attached to the sacrum at the lumbar sacral joint.

Fig. 1.1 Joints of the pelvis - Anterior view of pelvis with lumbar vertebrae

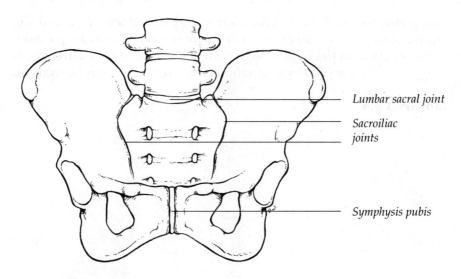

Lumbar sacral joint

Sacroiliac joints

Symphysis pubis

The pelvis protects the abdominal viscera, gives muscle attachments and transmits weight to the lower limbs.

The bones of the pelvis are held together by **ligaments** made of strong fibrous tissue consisting of fibroblasts and tightly packed bundles of collagen fibres. These ligaments give stability to the joints and counteract extreme or unexpected movements.

The ligaments are normally limited in their flexibility in order to protect the joints. During pregnancy, hormonal influence gives more pliability to these supporting tissues (see Ch. 2), leading to slightly increased movements in the joints of the pelvis and increased instability. This may cause pain and discomfort during pregnancy (see Ch. 2), and during the postnatal period (see Ch. 8). However, the "give" of these joints can produce additional space and thus increase the transverse and antero-posterior diameters of the pelvic outlet, which will be of advantage during labour and delivery.

It has been observed radiologically that there is an increase of 28% in the area of the pelvic outlet when the squatting position is used compared with the supine position *(Russell, 1982)*.

Anatomical relations

The abdominal cavity extends from the diaphragm down to the pelvic floor. Within the pelvic area of the cavity, the uterus and the vagina lie between the bladder and the urethra in front and the rectum and anus behind. The uterus projects into the vagina almost horizontally when a woman is in the standing position. It is held in position by ligaments and, indirectly, by the pelvic floor and is movable, for example, when a full bladder pushes it into a vertical position. During pregnancy the uterus enlarges and its position changes. It rises out of the pelvis and the upper part reaches the sternum by about 36 weeks gestation. During the last month of pregnancy the level falls when the fetal head descends into the pelvis. The growing uterus puts pressure on the bladder and bowel, which can lead to increased urinary frequency and intestinal discomfort.

Fig. 1.2 The pelvis showing the ligaments

a) Anterior view

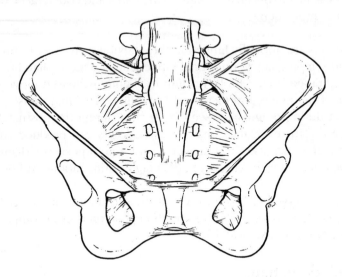

b) Posterior view

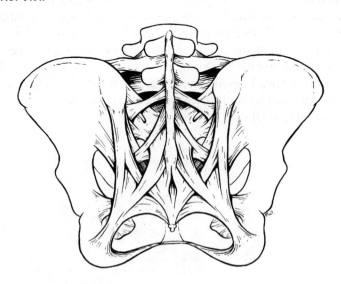

ABDOMINAL MUSCLES

The abdominal wall can be likened to a human corset and it is comprised of four sets of muscles and fascia on each side of the body. Three of these are flat muscles arranged in layers covering the anterior and lateral areas of the trunk. The fibres of each muscle end in an aponeurosis - a flat thin tendon which spreads out in the form of a broad sheet; most of the anterior abdominal wall is aponeurotic rather than muscular. The flat abdominal muscles are the **transversus abdominis** and the **internal and external oblique**. The fourth set, the **rectus abdominis**, is a band-like muscle lying on either side of the **linea alba** anteriorly. The linea alba is a fascial thickening in the midline, extending from the ziphoid process down to the pubic symphysis below.

The deepest muscle, the **transversus abdominis**, arises from the thoracolumbar fascia, the iliac crest and the inguinal ligament and above from the inner surface of the costal cartilages of the six lower ribs, interdigitating with the origin of the diaphragm. The muscle fibres run mainly horizontally forwards and end in an aponeurosis which takes part in the formation of the rectus sheath (described later) and then attaches itself to the length of the linea alba.

Fig. 1.3 Transversus abdominis

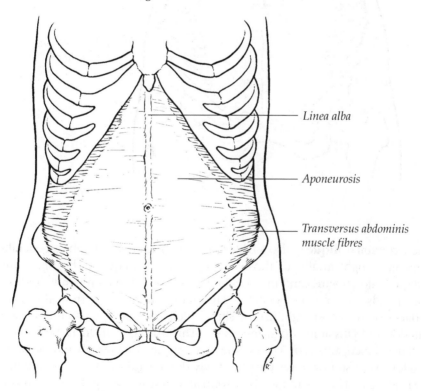

Linea alba

Aponeurosis

Transversus abdominis
muscle fibres

The **internal oblique** is a broad thin sheet lying between the transversus and the external oblique. It arises from the thoracolumbar fascia, the iliac crest and the inguinal ligament. It runs mainly upwards and forwards and the highest posterior fibres are inserted into the cartilages of the lower three ribs. The rest of the muscle fibres spread out and become an aponeurosis. This again takes part in the formation of the rectus sheath and then is attached to the xiphoid process, 7th, 8th and 9th costal cartilages, costal margin, linea alba and pubic crest.

Fig. 1.4 Internal oblique

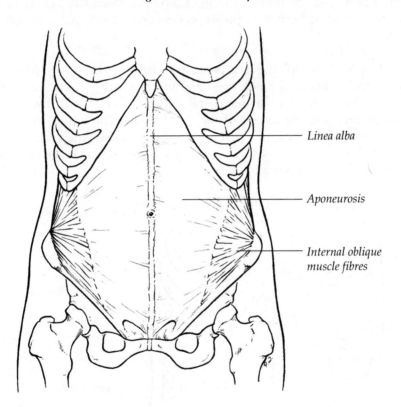

Linea alba

Aponeurosis

Internal oblique
muscle fibres

The **external oblique** is also a wide thin sheet of muscle with fibres generally running at right angles to those of the internal oblique. The fibres run obliquely downwards and inwards in the direction in which you would put your hands into trouser pockets. The muscle fibres arise from the outer surfaces of the lower eight ribs by slips which interdigitate with the serratus anterior and latissimus dorsi muscles. (This arrangement may be seen in well-developed subjects). The muscle fibres radiate downwards and forwards. The lowest posterior fibres pass vertically downwards and are inserted into the iliac crest. The rest of the fibres form an extensive triangular aponeurosis which is attached to the anterior superior iliac spine, the pubic tubercle and crest and the linea alba. The lower margin of the external oblique aponeurosis is folded back on itself between the anterior superior iliac spine and the pubic tubercle and forms the tendinous inguinal ligament. The anterior part of the aponeurosis helps to form the rectus sheath.

Fig. 1.5 External oblique

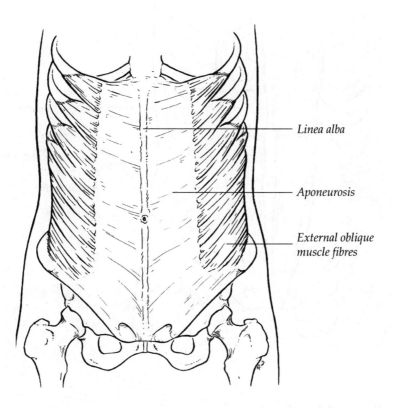

Linea alba

Aponeurosis

External oblique
muscle fibres

The most anterior and superficial of the abdominal muscles is the **rectus abdominis**. The muscle is long and strap-like and is located on either side of the midline. It is attached to the outer anterior part of the ribcage, the anterior aspect of the 5th, 6th and 7th costal cartilages and the xiphoid process. The muscle narrows as the fibres pass straight down the abdomen to divide into two tendons. The medial head is attached to the ligaments in front of the symphysis pubis, many of the fibres attaching themselves to the opposite side. The lateral head is attached to the pubic crest of its own side.

On the anterior surface of the muscle, but not extending through the entire substance of the muscle, are three (or more) transverse tendinous intersections at and above the umbilicus, which are firmly adherent to the anterior wall of the muscle sheath. These may be seen as transverse grooves on well-developed muscular male subjects.

Fig. 1.6 Rectus abdominis

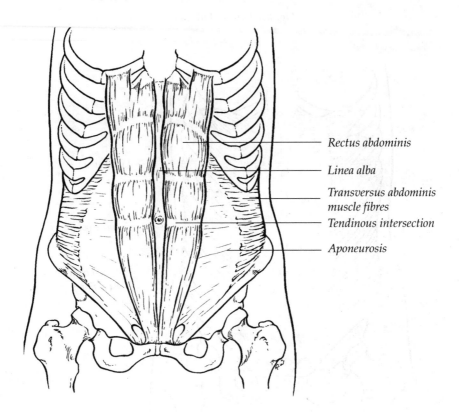

- Rectus abdominis
- Linea alba
- Transversus abdominis muscle fibres
- Tendinous intersection
- Aponeurosis

The Rectus Sheath

The rectus abdominis is wrapped in an envelope of fascia derived from the aponeuroses of the other abdominal muscles - the **rectus sheath**. The external oblique passes in front of the rectus sheath, the internal oblique separates to enclose it and the transversus abdominis passes behind. The sheath can stretch lengthways but less so crossways. Above the costal margin (see Fig. 1.7a), only the anterior wall of the sheath is present; it is made up entirely by the external oblique aponeurosis. Posteriorly, the rectus lies on the ribs and intercostal muscles. In the lower part of the abdomen (see Fig.1.7b), all three aponeuroses lie over the front of the rectus, the posterior wall being formed only by the fascia which lines the inside of the abdominal wall.

Fig. 1.7 Cross section through the rectus sheath

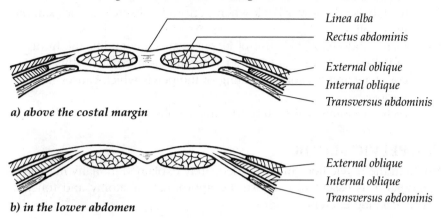

Linea alba

Rectus abdominis

External oblique
Internal oblique
Transversus abdominis

a) above the costal margin

External oblique
Internal oblique
Transversus abdominis

b) in the lower abdomen

A small triangular muscle, the **pyramidalis**, lies inside the rectus sheath, in front of the lower part of the rectus. It originates from the anterior surface the pubis and attaches itself to the linea alba. Its action is to tighten the linea alba. Pyramidalis is not always present and its absence may be implicated in diastasis seen below the umbilicus *(Boissonnault and Kotarinos, 1988)*.

The posterior abdominal wall is formed partly by the **quadratus lumborum**. This muscle originates from the iliac crest, the iliolumbar ligament and the transverse processes of the lower two or three lumbar vertebrae. It is attached to the inferior border of the 12th rib and the transverse processes of the upper two or three lumbar vertebrae.

Nerve supply

The lower six thoracic nerves supply the abdominal muscles. The oblique and transversus muscles are also supplied by the iliohypogastric and ilioinguinal nerves. The 2nd and 3rd lumbar nerves supply quadratus lumborum.

Functions of the abdominal muscles:

-   to support the abdominal contents in position partly by mechanical action and partly by maintaining intra-abdominal pressure.
-   to assist in control of posture; in partnership with the hip and back extensors, they control the tilt of the pelvis.
-   to increase, when all the abdominal muscles contract together, the intra-abdominal pressure and thus assist with all expulsive efforts such as coughing, micturition, defaecation, vomiting and parturition.
-   to effect movements of the trunk-flexion, side flexion and rotation,

- to brace the body when under stress, for example during lifting.
- to stabilise the lower back when performing exercises, for example knee-rolling.
- rectus abdominis, because of its pubic attachment, lifts the front of the pelvis (working together with gluteus maximus), thus counteracting the forward tilting of the pelvis which causes lumbar lordosis.
- rectus abdominis also supports the symphysis pubis.

THE PELVIC FLOOR

Although the pelvic floor may be adequately explained in many midwifery textbooks, it is essential to revise the appropriate anatomy and function before teaching exercise.

The pelvic floor forms a base to the pelvis and is composed of the **superficial perineal muscles**, fascia and the deeper **levator ani and coccygeus muscles**.

Superficial perineal muscles consist of small thin bands of striated muscle radiating outwards to the pelvic bones from the central tendinous perineal body. Each is one of a pair arising from each side.

Fig. 1.8 Superficial pelvic-floor muscles

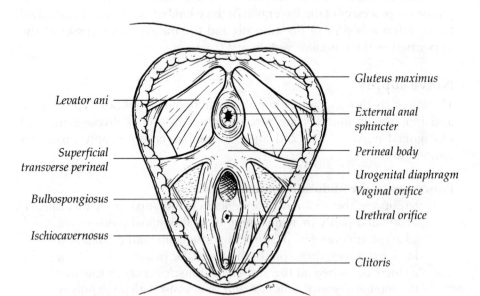

Levator ani

Superficial transverse perineal

Bulbospongiosus

Ischiocavernosus

Gluteus maximus

External anal sphincter

Perineal body

Urogenital diaphragm

Vaginal orifice

Urethral orifice

Clitoris

- **Bulbospongiosus** is attached to the perineal body round the vagina to the clitoris.
- **Ischiocavernosus** is attached to the ischial tuberosity and clitoris.
- **Superficial transverse perineal** attach the ischial tuberosities to the perineal body.
- **External anal sphincter** surrounds the anal orifice and is embedded in front of the perineal body and attaches itself behind the coccyx.

Fascia

A double sheet of fascia - the urogenital triangle or urogenital diaphragm - fills the triangular space below the symphysis pubis and the pubic rami. It is perforated in the middle to give passage to the vagina and urethra. The fascia also envelops the levator ani. It contains a few muscle fibres, namely the **compressor urethrae** and the **deep transverse perineal**. The latter is attached to the perineal body and helps to support and stabilise it. The fascia envelops and gives attachment to the muscles and is liable to be very stretched during childbirth. Muscles can be re-educated but fascia cannot.

Levator ani

This deep layer of muscles can be considered as one sheet of muscle and is covered by fascia; it forms a strong sling supporting the abdominal viscera. The muscles can be divided into the **iliococcygeus, pubococcygeus** and **puborectalis** and are attached to the pelvic surface of the pubic bone, obturator internus fascia and pelvic surface of the ischial spine. The muscle fibres pass with varying degrees of obliquity across the side of the vagina to be attached in the perineal body. The medial puborectalis fibres run either side of the urethra and vagina before being inserted into the perineal body, and the lateral fibres on each side encircle the rectum and blend with the external anal sphincter.

Fig. 1.9 Deep pelvic floor muscles

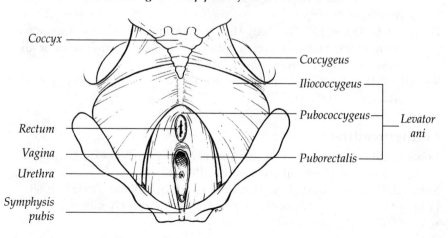

Coccygeus is a small triangular muscle which is posterior and superior to, but in the same plane as, the levator ani. It arises from the ischial spine and attaches itself onto the coccyx and lower sacrum.

The levator ani is composed of voluntary striated muscles incorporating type 1 (slow twitch) and type 2 (fast twitch) fibres *(Gosling et al., 1981)*. Type 1 fibres do not tire easily but the strength of the contraction is low. Type 2 fatigue easily but produce a high-strength contraction. So the levator ani can maintain tone and endurance, and can also resist sudden rises in abdominal pressure, for example on coughing or sneezing. So fast-twitch fibres work reflexly to "catch the cough".

Nerve supply
The above muscles are supplied by the pudendal plexus formed from the 2nd, 3rd, 4th and sometimes 5th sacral nerve routes (S2 - 5).

Functions of the Pelvic Floor:
  – it forms a base to the outlet of the pelvis.
  – it supports the pelvic organs.
  – it counteracts changes in abdominal pressure caused by such actions as coughing and lifting.
  – it assists in maintaining continence (urinary and faecal).
  – it produces a gutter to assist in the rotation of the fetal head during delivery.
  – it increases sexual enjoyment during intercourse.

The above functions are only performed efficiently if the muscles involved are maintained in a strong condition.

REFERENCES

Boissonnault J.S., Kotarinos R.K. Diastasis Recti. In: Wilder E., Ed., *Obstetric and Gynecologic Physical Therapy*. Edinburgh: Churchill Livingstone, 1988.

Gosling J.A., Dixon J.S., Critchley H.O.D., Thompson S. A comparative study of the human external sphincter and periurethral levator ani muscles. *Brit. J. Urol.*. 1981;53:35

Russell J.G.B. The Rationale of Primitive Delivery Positions. *Brit. J. Obstet. Gynaecol.*, 1982; 89:712

Further reading

Bennett V.R., Brown L.K., Eds. *Myles' Textbook for Midwives*. 12th Edn. Edinburgh: Churchill Livingstone. 1993.

Sweet B.R. *Mayes Midwifery*. 11th Edn. London: Ballière Tindall. 1988.

Polden M., Mantle J. *Physiotherapy in Obstetrics and Gynaecology*. Oxford: Butterworth-Heinemann. 1990.

CHAPTER 2

Physiological Changes and Minor Physical Problems in Pregnancy

Extensive physical and physiological alterations take place in a woman's body during pregnancy. These create challenges which should never be minimised.

THE RESPIRATORY SYSTEM

The changes to the respiratory system during pregnancy are both physiological and mechanical. The demand for oxygen is increased because the basal metabolic rate is raised as is the mass of the woman. At term the amount of oxygen required is about 20% above normal. There is a similar increase in the amount of carbon dioxide exhaled. The higher level of progesterone increases the sensitivity of the respiratory centre in the medulla to carbon dioxide levels in the blood *(Dale and Mullinax, 1988)*. This brings about a slight increase in the respiratory rate and there is a reduction of about 25% in the maternal blood carbon dioxide tension. Since the respiratory centre responds not to a scarcity of oxygen but to a surfeit of carbon dioxide, it is this lowering of the level of carbon dioxide which causes pregnant women to become breathless on activity. They often complain of difficulty in breathing (dyspnoea) even early in their pregnancies *(Patterson and Lindsay, 1988)*. There is a gradual increase in tidal volume by up to 40%. However, since the vital capacity remains more or less unchanged, there is an increase in ventilation of the alveoli due to a reduction in the volume of residual air.

Pregnant women may also hyperventilate *(Bush, 1992)*. This often happens during labour due to voluntary or involuntary overbreathing. Carbon dioxide is exhaled too forcefully leading to lightheadedness, tingling in the lips, hands and feet, sweating, panic and anxiety. Later symptoms could include unconsciousness. Theoretically, maternal hyperventilation could affect the fetus. The symptoms can be relieved and the condition reversed if the woman breathes with her cupped hands (or a paper bag) over her nose and mouth, thus re-inhaling her exhaled carbon dioxide. This will restore the blood gases to their normal level. The teacher should be aware of the risks of hyperventilation and unpleasant side effects, and teach ways of avoiding it. Practice of breathing awareness for labour should be done with breaks interspersed to prevent this occurring (see Ch. 5).

In many pregnant women the ascending uterus progressively obstructs the descent of the diaphragm. It may even force the diaphragm upwards by 4 cm or more towards the end of pregnancy *(Polden and Mantle, 1990)*. This upward pressure may also push the rib cage out sideways and forwards; stretching of the pliable tissues of the costal joint results in rib-flare. The antero-posterior and transverse diameters increase by about 10 cm *(Revelli et al., 1992)*. Rib-flaring can give rise to pain and discomfort along the anterior margin of the lower ribs (see page 25). Occasionally there is associated thoracic back pain. The flaring results in greater movements in the mid costal and apical regions of the chest. For this reason women often experience dyspnoea (breathlessness) even during mild exertion towards the end of their pregnancy.

THE CARDIOVASCULAR SYSTEM

The changes which occur in the cardiovascular system are impressive because they take place during a short space of time and there is complete restoration to the normal state after delivery.

The woman's blood volume increases by at least 40%. The plasma volume rises to a higher level than the red cell mass, causing the haemoglobin level to fall to about 12g/l *(Polden and Mantle, 1990)*. The resultant dilution anaemia may be one of the reasons why women feel tired from the early weeks of pregnancy.

The heart is pushed upwards by elevation of the diaphragm. It increases in size by about 12% *(Patterson and Lindsay, 1988)* due to stretching of the heart to accommodate the extra blood and to muscle hypertrophy. A recent study showed an increase in cardiac output from 4.9 to 7.2 litres/minute during pregnancy, the main rise being in the first trimester *(Robson et al., 1991)*. The rise in cardiac output is achieved mainly by increased heart rate with a small rise in stroke volume *(Chamberlain, 1991)*.

The smooth muscle of the walls of the blood vessels is relaxed by progesterone. This causes a small rise in body temperature and, more important, improves the peripheral circulation of the pregnant woman. Despite the increase in blood volume brought about by this hypotonia, blood pressure does not normally alter significantly during pregnancy. However, due to the slight decrease that may occur during the second trimester, women may feel faint when standing for too long. To avoid feeling dizzy, women should be reminded to take extra time when getting up from the lying position.

A pregnant woman may feel faint when lying on her back. This is due to the enlarging fetus compressing the aorta and inferior vena cava against the lumbar spine, and so restricting blood flow. This effect is known as pregnancy supine hypotensive syndrome and can be relieved by turning the woman onto her side and giving reassurance. Supine hypotension often occurs during the third trimester *(Revelli et al., 1992)*. However it has been suggested that it could occur after the fourth month of pregnancy *(Metcalfe et al., 1988)*. Teachers should be aware of this syndrome and would be wise to refrain from teaching exercise and relaxation in the supine position after the fourth month of pregnancy.

Varicosities and gravitational oedema may be brought about by various factors. These may include the increase of pressure within the abdomen caused by the enlarging uterus, the general increase of body weight, the slight reduction in vascular tone (brought about by progesterone) and changes in collagen structure (caused by progesterone and relaxin). Varicose veins of the legs and vulva and haemorrhoids may appear in pregnancy or, if already present, may be accentuated.

Late in pregnancy there may be oedema in the ankles, feet and hands which may lead to joint stiffness and nerve compression syndromes, the most common of which is carpal tunnel syndrome (see page 25).

THE MUSCULOSKELETAL SYSTEM
The changes which affect the musculoskeletal system are due primarily to the influence of the hormones oestrogen, progesterone and relaxin.

It is suggested that oestrogen prepares sites for the action of relaxin. Relaxin is produced as early as 2 weeks into pregnancy and is at its highest level in the first trimester, but then falls 20% *(Weiss, 1984)*, and remains at that level until delivery. Relaxin alters the composition of collagen, which is present in joint capsules, ligaments and fibrous connective tissue like the linea alba and intersections of the rectus abdominis muscle and the fascia of the pelvic floor. The remodelled collagen has greater elasticity and extensibility; the joints are therefore looser and the abdomen yields more. It has been suggested that, in a second pregnancy, the range of the joints is further increased but that in subsequent pregnancies no additional change is likely *(Calguneri et al., 1982)*. This laxity of the joints is gradually reduced after delivery, but the process may take up to 6 months before it is completed *(Polden and Mantle, 1990)*. The main joints affected by relaxin, and so especially vulnerable, are those of the pelvis. The symphysis pubis may separate - diastasis symphysis pubis (see page 24) and there can be increased movement in the sacroiliac joints. However, all joints are affected, the weight-bearing joints being especially susceptible to stress. Even the ligaments of the feet become lax and, with the additional weight of pregnancy, can cause discomfort. Pregnant women often complain of aching and flat feet. The costal inter-articular tissues become more pliable and permit the rib-flaring described earlier in this chapter.

As the uterus enlarges, the centre of gravity moves forwards and this causes the woman to alter her standing position. Her posture will depend on the strength of her muscles, her extra weight, laxity of her joints and tiredness. There is often exaggeration of the lumbar curve (lordosis) and compensatory curving of the thoracic spine (kyphosis). This can occur between the 4th and 9th months of pregnancy and persist until 12 weeks postnatally *(Bullock-Saxton, 1991)*. There may be rounding of the shoulders and protruding chin and the woman may lean back.

Fig. 2.1 a) Normal posture b) posture in pregnancy

a)

b)

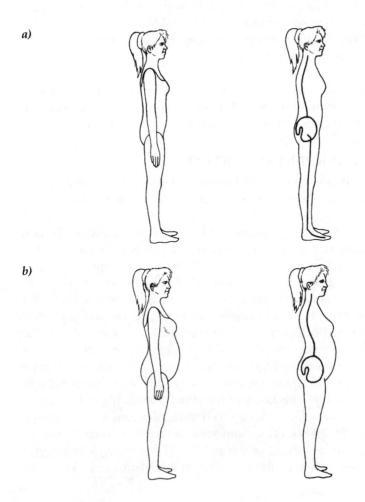

The incorrect posture imposes extra strain and fatigue on the body, particularly the spine, pelvis and weight-bearing joints and may give rise to aches and pains. In a study, Bullock *(1987)* found that 88.2% of women experienced back pain at some stage of their pregnancies. When questioned between 14 and 22 weeks gestation, 62% of the women reported that they had already experienced back pain. This suggests that abdominal enlargement was not the cause, but that hormonal changes and their influences on soft tissues may be important factors in producing the pain.

In a survey of 180 pregnant women, 48% reported significant backache. 15% of these considered the pain to be severe *(Mantle et al., 1977)*. Low back pain was often experienced, the pain sometimes spreading into the buttocks, the thighs and down the legs as sciatica. Sometimes there was also an increased tenderness over the symphysis pubis (see page 24). In a few women, the thoracic spine was similarly affected, the tenderness perhaps being caused in part by the increased size and weight of the breasts.

Additional pressure through the spinal column is caused by increased bodyweight, and stress to the joints results from increased torsion. The woman is often unbalanced and, the joints being more mobile, she is more prone to injury.

The abdominal wall has to adjust to accommodate the enlarging uterus and its muscle fibres stretch considerably. In a primigravida 162 cm tall the waistline can increase from 65 cm to 112 cm and the measurement from the xiphoid process to the symphysis pubis can increase from 39cm to 50 cm *(Polden, 1985)*. The linea alba, fibrous sheaths, aponeuroses and intersections are all composed of collagen and are made more supple by hormonal influence. The two muscles of the rectus abdominis separate as pregnancy advances. The intense stretching may even cause the linea alba to separate resulting in diastasis recti (see Ch. 7). The woman may experience a dragging, aching sensation in the lower abdomen as the weight of the uterus is transmitted through the abdominal muscles instead of those of the thighs. There may also be associated low-back pain. The strength of some muscles may actually increase during pregnancy as they have to support greater loads.

The enlarging uterus gradually increases pressure on the bladder and the smooth muscle of the bladder and the urethra can lose tone due to the influence of progesterone *(Chamberlain, 1991)*. It is also probable that the collagen present in the urethra and pelvic floor becomes more pliable. Hormonal action and increased weight during pregnancy can affect continence. It is suggested that in later pregnancy stress incontinence occurs in 50% of primigravidae and in nearly all multiparous women *(Francis, 1960, Jolleys, 1988)*.

With all these widespread changes in the woman's body, it is evident that the healthier and fitter she is both before and during pregnancy, the more easily she will cope with pregnancy. Ideally, she should prepare physically for each pregnancy and maintain good health while she is pregnant. Recovery after delivery should then be quicker. Exercises and advice are included in preparation for parenthood sessions (see Ch. 3), but some women will request alternative approaches to fitness, for example, exercise-to-music and aquanatal sessions (see Ch. 11).

SOME MINOR PHYSICAL PROBLEMS IN PREGNANCY

Cramp

Cramp is very common during pregnancy and especially affects the calf muscles. Its cause is not known. Circulatory exercises (see Ch. 3) often help in preventing attacks and are to be encouraged, especially before sleep as cramp often occurs at night. Stretching the leg and pointing the foot down (plantar flexion) often causes cramp so women must always remember to stretch with their feet pulled up (dorsiflexed). To alleviate cramp, the muscle should be put on a stretch by dorsiflexing the foot until the pain subsides.

Varicose veins

The varicose veins experienced by some women in pregnancy are caused by hormonal influence on the smooth muscle of the walls of the veins and the increased pressure within the abdomen. The circulatory exercises described in Chapter 3 should improve venous return. In severe cases, support tights may be recommended. To be effective these must be put on even before the woman swings her legs over the side of the bed, otherwise the veins will already be distended. Prolonged standing and sitting with feet down or legs crossed can aggravate the condition.

Diastasis symphysis pubis

Women with diastasis symphysis pubis will have pain and tenderness over the pubic area and down the inner thighs; the pain will vary in severity. Where possible the woman should be referred to an obstetric physiotherapist. If the condition is acute, bedrest with the legs held closely together (adducted) and slightly bent over a thin pillow or folded towel, is essential. The woman may require a supporting belt (ideally a trochanteric belt - see appendix) or girdle and, when the pain is less severe, she could wear this for doing light housework. She can be advised to keep her legs together when she rolls over and to take small shuffling steps when she walks to reduce the discomfort. She may need a walking frame or sticks for support. The medical notes must have clear instruction about this condition as special management in labour *(Fry, 1992)* will be required (see Ch. 5). Postnatal follow-up care by an obstetric physiotherapist should be given.

Carpal tunnel syndrome

Carpal tunnel syndrome is the most common nerve-compression syndrome. It is caused by compression of the median nerve as it passes though the carpal tunnel at the wrist. It usually occurs after about 24 weeks if there is marked fluid-retention. Some authors suggest that up to 50% of pregnant women have symptoms of this syndrome *(Melvin et al., 1969)*. Although it may be caused by localised oedema, it tends to be linked with generalised oedema. The woman often complains of numbness and stiffness in the fingers and she may find it difficult to pick up and hold small objects and to carry out small movements. This problem may be worse in the morning or at night when it may wake her up. Wrist-splints can often give relief at night and can be worn during the day as well if needed. In one survey, 46 out of 56 women became symptom-free by wearing wrist-splints at night *(Ekman-Ordeberg et al., 1987)*. The hands and arms should be supported in elevation when the woman is resting and she should be encouraged to perform wrist and hand exercises. Doing these in ice-cold water can sometimes give temporary relief. Women suffering from this condition should be warned to take extra care when handling hot liquids in a kettle, teapot or cup, especially first thing in the morning because they are more prone to accidents.

Rib-pain (Stitch)

Women often experience a stitch-like pain along the lower anterior and lateral ribs. It may be caused by rib-flaring or by the stretching of the abdominal muscles. The problem can often be relieved by clasping the hands and stretching the arms above the head. Side-bending slightly away from the pain with the arm and hand above the head may also help but care should be taken to avoid leaning very far to one side. Some women find reverse sitting astride a chair comfortable (see Ch. 5).

Stress incontinence

Stress incontinence is a frequent problem in pregnancy, especially during the third trimester. It should be discussed during antenatal classes and women reminded that assessment and treatment can be given if the condition continues postnatally. During pregnancy, regular exercising of the pelvic floor (see Ch. 3), should be encouraged; it is never too late to start. Women with more severe stress incontinence should be referred to an obstetric physiotherapist for individual assessment and treatment.

Tiredness (Fatigue)

Women often feel very tired during the first trimester and again in the last three months as they become heavier. Ideally they will need to cut down their workloads, their partners being reminded to help out more with household tasks. This can be discussed in couples sessions. Extra rest is essential and relaxation will be beneficial (see Ch. 4). Even if the woman is not complaining of tiredness, prevention is better than cure!

Low-back pain

The pregnant woman's weight has increased and she may be tired and so she may have poor posture. There is also instability of the joints caused by lax ligaments and the increased lumbar curve. These and several other factors can lead to low-back pain. If acute, the "first aid" would be bedrest in a comfortable position, possibly side-lying with the top leg resting on a pillow between the legs (see Fig.4.3, Ch 4). At home, the woman may find comfort by placing a hot water bottle wrapped in towels against her back. Where possible she should be referred to an obstetric physiotherapist for assessment and treatment.

When the pain is less severe, the woman can be shown gentle pelvic rocking (tilting). Advice should be given on such topics as positioning for rest, standing, walking and sitting posture, lifting, and advice on daily activities (see Ch. 3). The theme of back care should be continued postnatally (see Ch. 8).

The woman may need a back support, or a pantie-girdle may give some relief. Partners can be encouraged to try massage of the lower back as an aid to relaxation and the release of tension. Back-care advice (see Ch. 3) should be included as early as possible in the antenatal classes with the aim of preventing back pain *(Mantle, 1988)*.

REFERENCES

Bullock-Saxton J.E. Changes in posture associated with pregnancy and the early postnatal period measured in standing. *Physiotherapy Theory and Practice*, 1991;7:103

Bullock J.E., Jull G.A., Bullock M I. The relationship of low back pain to postural changes during pregnancy. *Austr. J. Physiotherapy*, 1987;33:10

Bush A. Cardiopulmonary effects of pregnancy and labour. *Journal of the Association of Chartered Physiotherapists in Obstetrics and Gynaecology*, 1992;71:3

Calguneri M., Bird H.A., Wright V. Changes in joint laxity occurring during pregnancy. *Ann. Rheum. Dis.*, 1982;41:126

Chamberlain G. The changing body in pregnancy. *Br. Med. J.*, 1991;302:719

Dale E., Mullinax K.M. Physiologic adaptations and considerations of exercise during pregnancy. In: Wilder E., Ed. *Obstetric and Gynecologic Physical Therapy*. Edinburgh: Churchill Livingstone, 1988.

Ekman-Ordeberg G., Salgeback S., Ordeberg G. Carpal tunnel tunnel syndrome in pregnancy. *Acta Obstet. Gynecol. Scand.* 1987;66:233

Francis W. The onset of stress incontinence. *J. Obst. Gynaecol. Br. Empire.* 1960;67:899

Fry D. Diastasis Symphysis Pubis. *Journal of the Association of Chartered Physiotherapist in Obstetrics and Gynaecology.* 1992;71:10

Jolleys J.V. Reported prevalence of urinary incontinence in women in a general practice. *Br. Med. J.* 1988;296:1300

Mantle M.J., Greenwood R.M., Currey H.L.F. Backache in pregnancy. *Rheum. Rehab.* 1977;16:95

Mantle M.J. Backache in pregnancy. In: McKenna J., Ed. *Obstetrics and Gynaecology.* Edinburgh: Churchill Livingstone, 1988.

Melvin J.L., Brunett C.N., Johnsson E.W. Median nerve conduction in pregnancy. *Arch. Phys. Med.* 1969;50:75

Metcalfe J., Stocks M.K., Barron D.H. Maternal physiology during gestation. In: Knobil E. & Neill J., Eds. *The Physiology of Reproduction.* New York: Raven Press, 1988.

Patterson C.A., Lindsay M.K. Maternal Physiology in Pregnancy. In: Wilder E., Ed. *Obstetric and Gynecologic Physical Therapy.* Edinburgh: Churchill Livingstone, 1988.

Polden M. Teaching Postnatal Exercises. *Midwives Cronicle & Nursing Notes.* 1985;10:271

Polden M., Mantle J. *Physiotherapy in Obstetrics and Gynaecology.* London: Butterworth - Heinemann, 1990.

Revelli A., Durando A., Massobrio M. Exercise and Pregnancy: A Review of Maternal and Fetal Effects. *Obstetrical and Gynecological Survey.* 1992;47(6):355

Robson S.C., Hunter S., Boys R. J., Dunlop W. Serial changes in haemodynamics during human pregnancy: a non-invasive study using Doppler echocardiography. *Clinical Science,* 1991;80:113

Weiss G. Relaxin. *Ann. Rev. Physiol.,* 1984;46:42

CHAPTER 3

Antenatal Exercises and Advice

In her book, *Safe Childbirth (1937)*, Dr Kathleen Vaughan described how her work with pregnant women who had led sedentary, inactive lives had shown that they frequently had difficult labours and deliveries. She recounted that for women of the Outer Hebrides who led laborious but healthy lives, and Kashmiri boatwomen and peasants, labour was easier. The way women used their bodies in everyday life had an important influence before, during and after childbirth.

Many exercise programmes were devised over the years *(Heardman, 1948, Randell, 1948, Wright, 1964, Madders, 1965, McLaren, 1978, Noble, 1978, Balaskas and Balaskas, 1979, Dale and Roeber, 1982)*. Despite the trend which some women follow towards continuing their chosen sport or activity into the later stages of their pregnancy, life for many is far less physically demanding than in the forties and fifties. Cars, washing machines and other present-day appliances have made life much easier physically.

It is important for a woman to maintain or improve her physical condition if she is to remain at her best throughout pregnancy and overcome the stresses placed upon her body by the development of the baby *(Hall and Kaufmann, 1987)*. Furthermore,having a healthy body during pregnancy helps to ensure a speedy recovery after the birth.

Advice should be offered about sport and other activities. Swimming and walking should be encouraged to help maintain cardiovascular and respiratory fitness and general body muscle tone and to relieve tension. The continuation of participation in competitive contact sports should be discouraged, and it is also inadvisable to start any new strenuous activity during pregnancy. However, for those women who wish to continue some fairly vigorous activity, antenatal exercise-to-music and/or aquanatal sessions would be a sensible alternative, provided these were led by fully qualified instructors (see Ch. 11). Moderate exercise has become the recommended formula for most mothers-to-be. Ideally women should increase their fitness prior to pregnancy. However, many attend early pregnancy sessions at 12-16 weeks or even 30 weeks into their pregnancy not having learned or tried any appropriate exercise programmes, although some may have read about them. Women frequently ask for exercises and it would therefore seem that a few carefully chosen exercises which are not too demanding should be incorporated into preparation for parenthood classes.

BASIC ANTENATAL EXERCISES

Circulatory exercises

Circulatory exercises should be practised frequently, particularly in the early morning and late evening; they should be performed in a sitting position with the legs elevated. They are intended to maintain and improve the circulation. Vigorous movements of the feet will assist venous return and minimise varicosities, swelling of the ankles and cramp.

Foot exercises

Sit or lie at an angle of 45 degrees (half-lying) with the back against a wedge and pillows, the legs supported and the knees straight. Bend and stretch the ankles briskly about 10 times, emphasising dorsiflexion rather than plantar flexion to avoid cramp. Keeping the knees and hips still, circle both ankles in as large a circle as possible 10 times in each direction.

Leg-tightening

Sit or lie (half-lying) in the same position as above. Pull both feet upwards at the ankle and press the back of the knees down onto the support. Hold this position for a count of 4, breathing normally, then relax. Repeat 5 times.

Fig. 3.1 Foot exercises

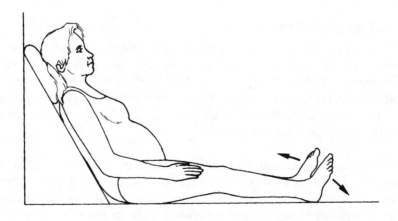

A pregnant woman should be advised to avoid prolonged standing, and sitting or lying with her legs crossed. She should be encouraged to sit with her legs supported horizontally. If oedema is present, she could lie at an angle of 45 degrees with her legs raised a little higher than her hips. It is important to retain a wide angle at the groin in order to prevent compression which could cause circulatory stasis.

Fig. 3.2 *Legs elevated in a half-lying position*

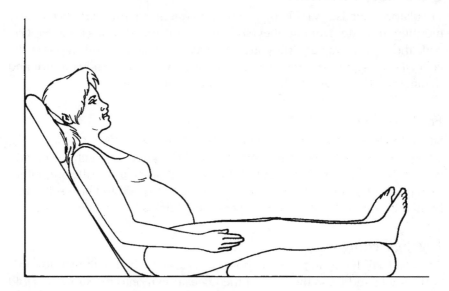

Sitting instead of standing must be encouraged and the woman reminded that walking will also aid her circulation. She should be advised to wear good supporting footwear and avoid high heels which might cause injury through instability.

Pelvic-floor exercises

Pelvic-floor exercises should receive top priority in any programme of physical exercise during pregnancy. Muscles toned antenatally will be able to cope with the stresses and strains put on them by pregnancy and to give extra support to the relaxing fascial layer. The woman will also understand more easily how to re-educate them after delivery; this will help to prevent any long-term urinary problems or prolapse.

Pelvic-floor exercises should definitely be taught, even late in pregnancy. Healthy, exercised muscles stretch and recoil more easily, which can facilitate delivery. It has been shown that pelvic-floor muscles are stronger postnatally in women who exercised during pregnancy than in those who did not (*Nielsen, 1988*).

Ideally women will have been introduced to pelvic-floor exercise before pregnancy, but many women will not have heard of it. The exercise should be started as early as possible in pregnancy. Before the exercise is taught, the relevant anatomy and the importance of these muscles must be explained in simple terms. A model pelvis and drawings will be helpful.

Pelvic-floor exercise

The pelvic-floor exercise can be practised in any comfortable position as long as the legs are slightly apart, not crossed.

Close the back passage as though preventing a bowel action, close the middle and front passages too as though preventing the flow of urine, then lift up all three passages inside. Hold strongly for as long as possible up to 10 seconds, breathing normally throughout. Relax and rest for 3 seconds. Repeat **slowly** as many times as you can, up to a maximum of 10. Repeat the exercise, this time lifting up and letting go **more quickly** up to 10 times without holding the contraction.

By exercising these muscles slowly and quickly, both the slow-twitch and fast-twitch muscle fibres will be activated *(Gilpin et al., 1989)*. A reliable schedule for the exercise may be provided by linking them to daily activities, for example washing up, **after** each bladder-emptying, or by displaying stickers around the house.

Time must be given in the session for questions and discussion to help the women to try out the exercise and to understand it thoroughly. Some may need further advice in order fully to appreciate the feeling and to be confident that they can contract the muscles. Chiarelli *(1991)* states that it might prove dangerous to use the urine "stop and start" mechanism as an exercise, as this practice is not good bladder-training. However, a mid-stream stop could be used as an occasional test, preferably on the second or subsequent voiding of the day.

More time should be afforded during the following sessions to recapitulate and offer further guidance. Another way to recognise the contractions might be by observation in a mirror when squatting. Gripping the penis during intercourse, thus sharing the exercise with the partner, can have the benefit of feed-back.

Women should be advised to contract the pelvic floor when coughing, sneezing, laughing, lifting or squatting.

Abdominal exercises

As pregnancy progresses, the pelvis tends to be tilted further forwards. This puts stress on the ligaments and joints of the lower back and pelvis which could lead to pain and discomfort. Pelvic tilting is an exercise chosen for preventing and relieving back pain and stiffness and for promoting good posture. The exercise also works the abdominal muscles and hip extensors and helps to maintain their tone. These muscles will offer support and protection to the pelvic joints and lower back as the ligaments become more supple.

Pelvic tilting

Lie at an angle of 45 degrees (half-lying) supported by a wedge and pillows, with the knees bent and the feet flat on the surface. Pull in the abdominal muscles, tighten the muscles of the buttocks and press the small of the back down onto the support. Hold the position for a count of 4, breathing normally, then relax. Repeat 5 times. The exercise may also be performed more rhythmically to help relieve any tension and postural backache whenever the need arises.

Fig. 3.3 Pelvic tilting in a half-lying position with the knees bent up

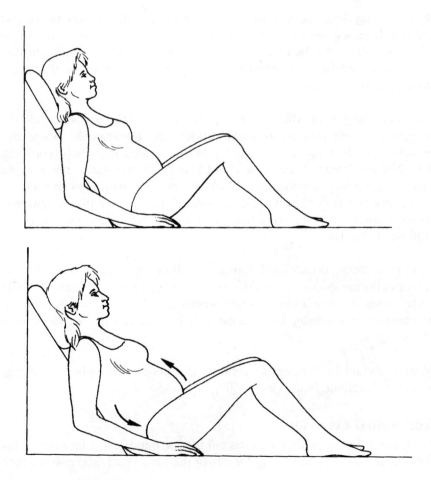

Once mastered in the above position, pelvic tilting can be encouraged in several positions, for example sitting, reverse sitting, side-lying, standing against a wall, standing looking into a mirror sideways, supported kneeling and prone kneeling*. It may be practised slowly at least two or three times a day and, as with the pelvic-floor exercise, it can be performed in conjunction with many daily activities.

* Prone-kneeling is often a favourite position for practising pelvic tilting. However, the abdominal muscles are working against gravity and the back tends to hollow putting stress on the lower back. Care should be taken to start in a neutral position (back flat - not hollow) and return to the starting position slowly. Partners can check that performance is correct and discourage sagging of the spine.

Fig. 3.4 Pelvic tilting in prone kneeling position

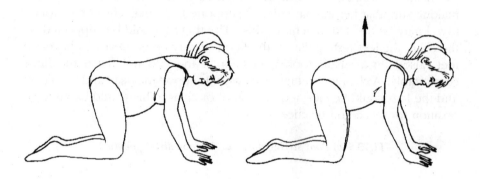

Abdominal retraction

Lie at an angle of 45 degrees (half-lying) supported by a wedge and pillows, with the knees bent, or sit or stand. Pull in the abdominal muscles. Hold them in for a count of 4, breathing normally, then relax. Repeat 5 times. This can be performed frequently in any position, with or without the pelvic tilt. Bracing the abdominal muscles is a safe, simple exercise which also helps to tone the muscles.

BACKCARE DURING PREGNANCY

The body, whether it is stationary or moving, should be respected at all times. However, this is especially important during pregnancy and for many months following delivery. During these times, the back and pelvic area are particularly vulnerable (see Ch. 2). To prevent long-term back problems and strain on stretched muscles, extra consideration must be given to the back when sitting, lifting, bending and moving and in household activities and/or in working positions at the office or other place of employment.

The midwife will need to explain the relevant anatomy and physiology to women and their partners and discuss possible problems. A ligamented model pelvis is very helpful to illustrate joints and vulnerable areas. In antenatal classes, small groups of women and partners can be asked to consider positions, movements and tasks which could lead to problems. This, followed by a whole-group feedback and discussion, is an interesting way of covering this topic.

Heavy, strenuous work should be avoided. Rather than risking pain and tiredness, help should be asked for. However, guidance and advice on how she might adapt and modify daily activities can allow the woman to continue many of her commitments well into pregnancy.

Sitting

Sitting is a commonly adopted position, so good posture and comfort are essential. A woman needs to be reminded to sit well back in her chair making sure that her lumbar spine is supported. A small cushion or rolled towel may be needed to achieve this. The thighs should be supported by the chair, the feet resting flat on the floor. It may be necessary to have the feet raised on a small stool or cushion if they do not reach the floor comfortably. A chair with a high back would support the head and shoulders and the legs could be elevated on a stool or chair. This would be an ideal position for relaxation practice.

Fig. 3.5 a) Poor sitting posture   b) good sitting posture

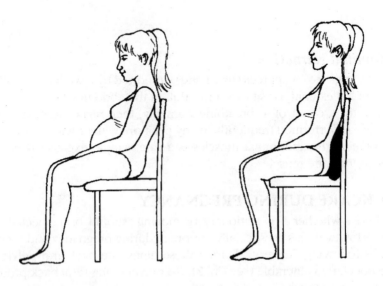

Standing

The aspects of good upright posture must be discussed. The woman needs to be encouraged to stand and "walk tall", pulling the abdominal muscles in and tucking the buttocks under so the pelvis is tilted back. The position of the head is important - it should be held high with the chin tucked in and with shoulders down and relaxed. It might be suggested that the woman imagines a thread pulling her up to the ceiling from the head - to "think tall" and stretch out the spine. Alternatively she could be asked to try to stretch between the hips and the ribs to make more room for the baby. This will lessen the curves and so reduce the muscular effort used during standing. In order to keep good balance, the feet should be apart with the body weight distributed evenly through both legs and down through the outer border of each foot.

Standing still for too long can lead to tiredness and strain. So it is better to walk around but it is important that all the points of good, upright posture should be maintained. The woman should "listen to her body" and not walk for too long as this can lead to discomfort.

Fig. 3.6 Poor and good posture in standing

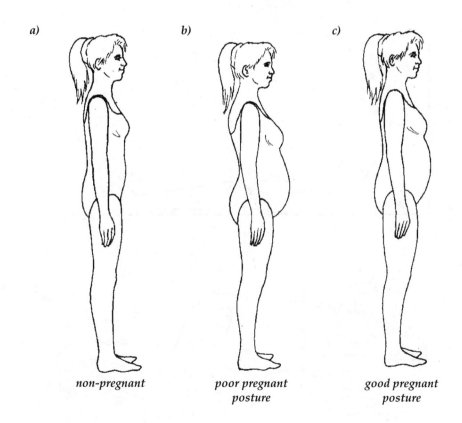

a)   b)   c)

non-pregnant   poor pregnant   good pregnant
                           posture   posture

Lying

Because of the risk of supine hypotension, lying flat on the back should be discouraged after the fourth month of pregnancy (see Ch. 2). If the supine position is used in early pregnancy, a pillow under the thighs gives extra comfort. As pregnancy advances, the woman usually finds more difficulty in getting comfortable because of the increase in her size and weight. It is important that she alters her position and is well supported giving equal pressure on all parts of the body in order to get rest and sleep and to prevent strain. For back-lying, extra pillows or a wedge will raise the head and shoulders enough and a pillow under the thighs will prevent stretch on the lower back and knees. Most women prefer side-lying or three-quarters-lying position with two pillows under the head and one under the top knee and thigh to prevent strain on the sacroiliac joint. A small cushion or rolled towel may add to comfort if placed under the waist or abdomen, especially if the mattress is not very firm. If side-lying is chosen, an extra pillow should be used to support the top forearm. Pain and strain at the symphysis pubis and sacroiliac joints can be minimised if the woman bends her knees up and keeps them pressed together when she turns over in bed.

Fig. 3.7 a) Half-lying, b) side-lying and c) three quarters-lying

a)

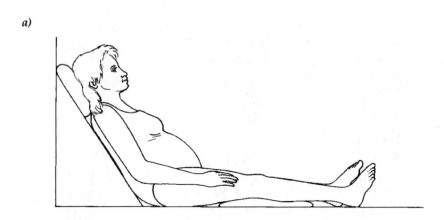

b)

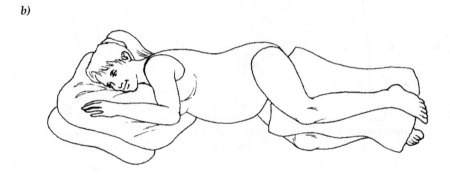

c)

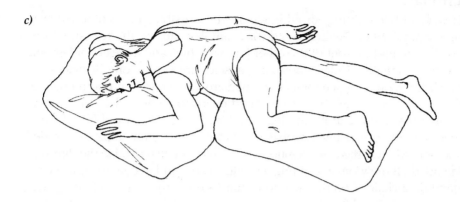

Getting up from the bed or examination couch should be demonstrated to the group and practised. Both knees must be bent and kept together, the whole body rolled over to one side and then pushed up into the sitting position using the upper hand and lower elbow, with the legs now over the side of the bed. The woman slowly stands up, straightening her legs. This is done in reverse when getting onto a bed or couch. Midwives need to encourage this care in antenatal clinics, not only to protect the back, but also the abdominal muscles. Sitting straight up forwards is similar to performing a sit-up exercise and must be discouraged. When rising from the floor, the woman should go over on her hands and knees and then push herself up onto one knee using the opposite arm for support. She then pushes herself up into the standing position by slowly straightening her legs. This again requires demonstration and practice.

Fig. 3.8 Getting up from lying

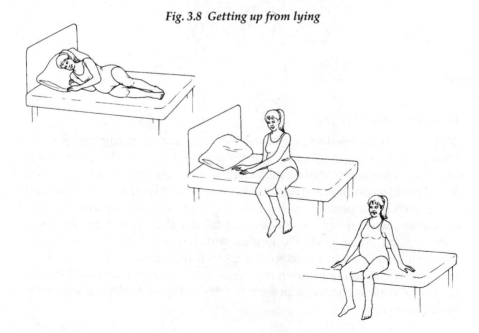

37

Lifting

Heavy, difficult lifting should, whenever possible, be avoided during pregnancy. When having to lift, for example toddlers, the feet should be apart - one foot in front of the other - and the hips and knees bent keeping the back straight. Unless the thigh muscles are very strong, it places too much strain on the knee joints if women are advised to bend both knees to their full extent. The object to be lifted needs to be held close and central to the body and the arms and legs used for lifting. This would be done in reverse to put down a heavy object. Twisting when lifting must be avoided and only when in the erect position should the feet be moved in the direction intended. If the woman is lifting a toddler, she could encourage him/her to stand on a chair or on the second or third step of the stairs so that she can avoid stooping to lift.

Fig. 3.9 Correct lifting

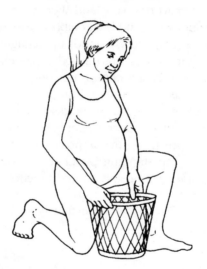

Household activities

Women can be advised to perform housework in an easy, rhythmical way - avoiding jerky movements, so putting less strain on the body and avoiding tiredness. Vacuuming must be performed in a straight line, avoiding twisting as this could stress the sacroiliac joints. Working levels need to be checked to maintain good posture - a high stool can prevent leaning and possible backache. Women can be encouraged to sit rather than stand for some tasks. Sitting down to do the ironing with the board lowered would be ideal but getting accustomed to this takes some practice! Alternatively, if ironing in the standing position is preferred, the height of the board should be such as to allow comfort with the feet apart and space to move rhythmically from side to side.

When bathing toddlers, making beds, cleaning the bath or cuddling little ones, kneeling will prevent backache. Some women will be able to use the squatting position, with one knee in front of the other, when getting down to low cupboards or drawers or to cuddle, again preventing lumbar strain; others will prefer to kneel to avoid stooping.

Fig. 3.10 Kneeling to bath and cuddle toddler

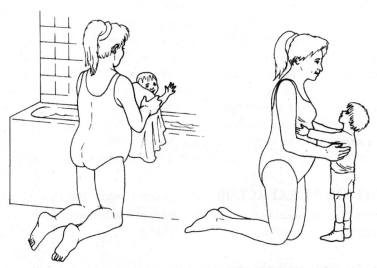

When shopping, women should keep the supermarket trolley close to the body and, ideally, load-carrying should be reduced to a minimum. If carrying the shopping, it can either be held close to the body or separated into two equal amounts for balanced transport.

Fig. 3.11 Carrying shopping

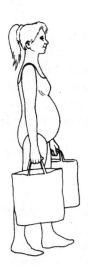

When getting into the car, sit first and then, tightening the abdominals and keeping the knees together, bring the legs round into the car; this should be performed in reverse when getting out. When driving, the back needs to be well supported. Care should be taken, when putting on the seat belt and when reversing, to avoid twisting round in a jerky way.

Care of the back is an essential topic for inclusion in antenatal sessions with discussion and demonstrations. It is important to try to prevent problems before they arise and cause pain. For this reason, consideration of baby equipment and care in relation to backs and safety should be covered. It can be especially interesting for topics such as nappy-changing and bathing to be discussed with women when partners are present. They should realise that activities need to be stopped **before** pain is felt. Helping the women and partners to recognise what could cause this pain, so learning body-awareness, will prevent problems. They should be reminded that the more often a **correct** movement (e.g.lifting) is performed, the more likely the performance will become an automatic, learned pattern of movement.

ADDITIONAL EXERCISES (instructions can be found in Chapter 9)

These may be included in conventional preparation for parenthood sessions and are:

Shoulder, arm and chest exercises

Women often ask for exercise for the "breasts". The breast tissue is not muscle and therefore cannot be exercised. However, shoulder and chest exercises (see Ch. 9) could improve circulation and comfort in the area and working the pectoral muscles may offer support for the breasts. Women should also be encouraged to wear a good supporting bra.

Stretching exercises

The muscles and ligaments of the groin, hips and lower limbs (especially the adductors and calf muscles) will have shortened in many women, mainly due to our sedentary life style. Stretching exercises will help women to take up and hold various positions more comfortably during labour and delivery. The exercises prepare the women both physically and psychologically and encourage them to feel comfortable with wide-open legs, a position which they are not used to adopting.

EXERCISES TO AVOID

Two commonly practised "abdominal" exercises are double-leg raising and sit-ups with straight legs. These are very high risk exercises for anyone to perform and may result in compression injury to vertebral discs and muscle and ligament damage *(Donovan et al., 1988)*. There are added risks to the pregnant woman because of stretched muscles and lax ligaments (see Ch.2).

Fig. 3.12 .Double-leg raising and sit-ups with straight legs

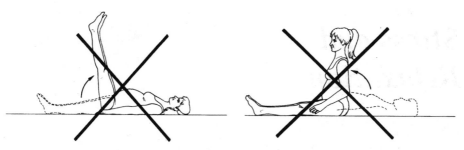

**THESE TWO EXERCISES SHOULD <u>NEVER</u> BE
PERFORMED DURING PREGNANCY**

References

Balaskas A., Balaskas J. *New Life*. London: Sidgwick & Jackson, 1979.

Chiarelli P.E. *Women's Waterworks: Curing Incontinence*. New South Wales: Gore & Osment Publishing Pty Ltd. 1991.

Dale B.,Roeber J. *Exercises for Childbirth*. London: Century Publishing, 1982.

Donovan G., McNamara J., Gianoli P. *Exercise Danger.* Western Australia: Wellness Australia Pty Ltd. 1988.

Gilpin S.A., Gosling J.A., Smith A.R.B., Warrell D.W. The pathogenesis of genitourinary prolapse and stress incontinence of urine. A histological and histochemical study. *Brit. J. Obstet. Gynaecol.* 1989;96:15

Hall D.C., Kaufmann D.A. Effects of Aerobic and Strength Conditioning on Pregnancy Outcomes. *Am. J. Obstet. Gynecol.* 1987;157:1199

Heardman H. *A Way to Natural Childbirth*. Edinburgh: E & S Livingstone Ltd, 1948.

Madders J. *Before and After Childbirth*. Edinburgh: E & S Livingstone Ltd., 1965.

McLaren J. *Preparation for Parenthood*. London: John Murray, 1978.

Nielsen C.A., Sigsgaard I., Olsen M., et al. Trainability of the pelvic floor. *Acta Obst. Gynecol. Scand.* 1988;67:437

Noble E. *Essential Exercises for the Childbearing Year (revised edn.)*. London: John Murray, 1982.

Randell M. *Fearless Childbirth*. London: Churchill, 1948.

Vaughan K. *Safe Childbirth*. London: Ballière Tindall & Cox, 1937.

Wright E. *The New Childbirth*. London: Tandem, 1964.

Further reading

Noble E. *Essential Exercises for the Childbearing Year, 3rd Edn.* Boston: Houghton Mifflin, 1988.

Williams M., Booth D. *Antenatal Education*. Edinburgh: Churchill Livingstone, 1985.

CHAPTER 4

Stress and Relaxation

Relaxation is a topic included in most preparation for parenthood courses as stated in the New Pregnancy Book (1993). Women and partners request its inclusion and they are therefore interested and motivated.

Most of us show some signs of tension when difficulties pile up. We feel tense, achy and tired and we even question whether we can cope. It is often a very insignificant incident which can turn out to be "the last straw" and which can finally "break the camel's back". We say that we are "uptight" or "under stress".

What is stress?

The stress of "modern day living", a popular phrase today, may be brought about by any situation which gives rise to anxiety, uneasiness, irritation, fear, frustration or even anger. In biological language, "stress" means anything which creates a threat, whether real or imaginary, which might adversely impinge upon an organism.

The body prepares for "fight or flight" whenever it seems to be threatened. This is a primitive animal instinct - an emergency reaction. However, in humans such reactions are produced not just when there is real danger, but also when there is no real threat to life at all. Unfortunately, it is this human inability to distinguish between the real and the imaginary threat which can eventually lead to stress disorders.

Some tension is necessary for performance but too much reduces achievement and leads to fatigue, pain and possibly illness. As soon as a threat is recognised, a reflex which short-cuts the brain is triggered. Muscles immediately tense for action ready in the fight-flight response. We assume the common posture of tension. In sitting,

- the head comes forwards
- the shoulders are elevated
- the elbows are flexed and kept close to the body
- the fists are clenched

42

- the legs are crossed with feet dorsiflexed
- the body is bent forwards and is usually rigid
- the facial expression is often one of worry with the jaw clamped tightly shut

This position of tension would be modified in standing or lying.

Fig. 4.1 Stress position

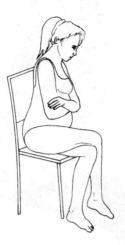

The danger message is received by the brain and internal responses are made. Dramatic changes in the working of the cardiovascular system become evident. The heart rate increases, the blood pressure rises and constriction of blood vessels in the skin and the digestive and reproductive systems results in diversion of blood to the brain, lungs and locomotor muscles. The respiratory system is also affected; breathing is either held on an inward gasp or becomes shallower and more rapid. The emphasis is on inspiration. Additionally, the mouth becomes dry, sweating increases and other more complicated changes occur.

When appropriate action has been taken and the danger is over, everything settles down to normal, relaxation takes place and no harm is done. It is when these normal and valuable reactions are prolonged, exaggerated and inappropriate that illness and disease can result.

Adopting the position of tension in itself causes increased tension and fatigue. Prolonged arousal can lead to others noticing the signs of strain such as grumbling, irritability, decreased achievement at work (although more time spent there!), increased smoking and drinking and inadequate sleep. It is at this stage that "the straw **will** break the camel's back".

Fig. 4.2 Effects of stress

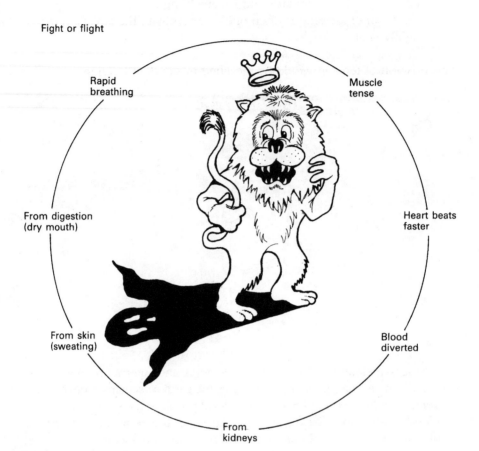

Fight or flight

Rapid breathing

Muscle tense

From digestion (dry mouth)

Heart beats faster

From skin (sweating)

Blood diverted

From kidneys

Stress in Pregnancy

The American psychiatrists, Drs. Holmes and Rahe (1967), devised a scale of various stressful events, pregnancy being high on the scale. In pregnancy, the woman's body is in a different and changing physiological condition which will affect not only her physical state but her psychological state too. She will have all the everyday stresses to which we are subjected plus the physical and emotional pressures that pregnancy brings. To mention but a few of these stresses:

- was the baby planned?
- will it be healthy?
- what is the mother's work situation?
- is she provided with adequate finance?
- has she a supportive partner?

She will also have the physical stresses of pregnancy to cope with:
- is she exhausted and feeling nauseous?
- has she aching joints?
- does she feel clumsy and less mobile?

Additionally, she may be anxious about labour and motherhood which will give rise to added tension.

The pregnant woman also shares the physical effects of her emotions with the fetus. If her feelings of anxiety are increased, especially if they are prolonged and extreme, they may affect her baby. The increased chemicals and hormones produced by the anxiety state circulate in the body and can cross the placenta and reach the fetus *(Madders, 1979)*. There may also be a relationship between a new baby's restlessness and extensive crying and a mother's emotional distress.

All the systems of the body are affected and the challenges these changes make on the pregnant woman should never be underestimated.

How can we cope with stress?

We can learn to understand ourselves, to realise how much we can put up with and to admit if we can't cope.
We should take time out for hobbies and leisure activities.
We should, if possible, "create some space" for ourselves.
We should eat well, exercise and keep fit.

We should recognise that relaxation can be an efficient way of dealing with stress. A state of muscle relaxation is incompatible with that of anxiety. A relaxed person cannot be anxious, nor when anxious, can be truly relaxed *(Woodrow, 1988)*.

RELAXATION TECHNIQUES

Progressive relaxation (the contrast method) was commonly taught in childbirth education classes. Dr Edmund Jacobsen outlined the technique which involved alternately contracting and relaxing muscle groups progressively throughout the body *(Jacobsen, 1938)*. From this, the woman learned to recognise the difference between relaxation and tension. Unfortunately, many using this method found that the body remained in a posture of tension, as those muscles which were tense were never lengthened - so the position of tension remained. Also, normal breathing was affected as breath-holding often took place as each muscle group was contracted.

Physiological relaxation is now the method more widely taught by obstetric physiotherapists and midwives. This was developed by Laura Mitchell in 1987 and is a simple, exact technique. If one group of muscles is contracted, the opposite muscle group is stretched (relaxed). Clear orders are given to the opposite group of muscles to work and so the muscles which were tense are compelled to relax. This method is based on the physiological principle of reciprocal relaxation. Muscles move the joints into a position of ease; this will be a "neutral" position. In her book, *Simple Relaxation,* Laura Mitchell points out that information about the state of relaxation or contraction of a muscle is not carried to the conscious brain - the brain only receives information about a muscle's movement. Proprioceptors in joints and muscle tendons and receptors in the skin register the resulting position of ease and this is communicated to the brain where it is recorded in the cerebrum. Clear and concise instructions are given to each area of the body affected by stress. Three instructions are used in a fixed order throughout the body and they result in body awareness of the posture of ease for relaxation.

The sequence of instructions for each joint is:
1.   **Move** into the position opposite to that of stress.
2.   **Stop** doing the movement.
3.   **Check** the new position of the joint and, if applicable, the skin sensation.

Fig. 4.3 Position of ease

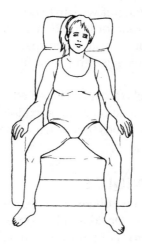

Relaxation for the pregnant woman and partner may be practised in any comfortable, supported position - sitting, lying and three-quarters-lying are often chosen at first. The recommended sequence for the relaxation is:-

1.   Arms
2.   Legs
3.   Body
4.   Head
5.   Face
6.   Breathing

1. Arms

Shoulders Pull your shoulders down towards your feet.
STOP pulling your shoulders down.
Feel that your shoulders are now lower and your neck feels longer.

Elbows Push your elbows slightly away from your side.
STOP pushing your elbows out.
Be aware that your elbows are open and slightly away from your side.

Hands Stretch out your hands, fingers and thumbs.
STOP stretching them out.
Observe that your hands, fingers and thumbs are fully supported.
Feel the surface on which they are resting.

2. Legs

Hips Roll your hips and knees outwards.
STOP rolling outwards.
Be aware that your legs are slightly apart and turned outwards.

Knees Adjust until comfortable.
STOP adjusting.
Reflect on the resulting position.

Feet Gently push your feet down, away from your face.
STOP pushing them down.
Feel your feet hanging loosely from the ankle joints.

3. Body

Press your body into the support.
STOP pressing.
Consider the sensation of your body resting against the support.

4. Head

Press your head into the pillow.
STOP pressing.
Feel your heavy head nestling comfortably in the hollow you have made in the pillow.

5. Face

Jaw Keeping your lips closed, pull down your lower jaw.
STOP pulling down.
Feel that your teeth are no longer touching and that the jaw-line is easy.

Tongue Move your tongue low in your mouth.
STOP moving.
Register that your tongue is lying in the middle of your mouth.

Eyes Close your eyes, if you wish to, or stare instead.

Forehead Imagine someone smoothing away your frown lines from the eye-brows up over the top and the back of your head.
STOP doing this.
Feel the smoothing of the skin.

6. Breathing

Sigh out Breathe low down in your chest at your own natural resting breathing rate, with slight emphasis on the out breath.

To prevent your brain being too active during your physical relaxation, concentrate on something pleasant and happy which helps you to feel comfortable. The whole sequence should be repeated probably a little quicker and then women and partners told how long they will be left to relax.

This deep relaxation is often referred to as passive relaxation. At the end of the period of relaxation, you should open your eyes and consider your position - how open and unfolded you are compared with the position of tension. Remember never to get up quickly following complete passive relaxation. The circulation needs to be stimulated by stretching and performing foot and hand movements before sitting up slowly. After a minute or two, full activity can be resumed. There is a very close link between relaxation and breathing. It is very difficult to allow breathing to be calm and flow easily if one is tense, and difficult to relax if breathing is forced or controlled. Women and partners should be encouraged to increase their awareness by linking the two in practice and then using them as coping skills for labour (see Ch. 5) and everyday stresses. Women should be encouraged to practise the relaxation technique every day of their pregnancy, either sitting supported in an arm chair whilst watching television, or lying on the bed for an afternoon rest or in bed before going to sleep. Relaxation practised during pregnancy will help to lower blood pressure *(Benson, 1988)*. Fatigue and tension will be relieved and so there will be fewer aches and pains. The woman will be less anxious and the baby will gain too! *(Madders, 1979)*.

Giving birth is, perhaps, the greatest athletic experience a woman is likely to take part in - both physically and emotionally. The woman may be fearful and anxious about the pain of labour, about her safety and that of her baby. For those delivering in the hospital, tension may be increased by the woman taking on a "patient" role. She may feel she will not have responsibility for her own labour and that she could lose control and dignity. In this respect, individuals vary enormously. To a lesser degree, the father may also have anxieties.

The "fight-flight" response will be made in response to pain, fear or apprehension and can lead to increased physical discomfort or pain and to inhibition of the uterine activity and dilatation of the cervix.

With practice, relaxation can be used as a coping skill for labour (see Ch. 5). Energy is conserved and blood pressure kept lower by practising passive relaxation of voluntary muscles between contractions. During contractions, active relaxation can be used to raise the pain threshold, to increase the endurance to pain and allow labour to progress more easily. In order for the woman (and partner) to be able to use the relaxation skill actively for labour, frequent practice is essential. As well as using comfortable positions for training, it is necessary to try out this skill using postures which may be used in labour (see Chapter 5.)

Relaxation can be used postnatally especially during disturbed nights or if the mother is anxious about coping with the new baby. It is also an aid to successful breastfeeding.

Before teaching relaxation, it is important for you to consider your attitude to this skill. Maybe you are only teaching it because you have to take your turn on the rota! Do **you** use it yourself? If not, should you begin to use it? Do you believe that it is an important coping technique for use in labour? Remember that your beliefs and views will filter through in your teaching however careful you try to be. You must have a full understanding of the method of relaxation you decide to teach - how it reduces tension and the value for the woman and partner during pregnancy, labour and the puerperium. Consider at what stage in your session you will include relaxation - it need not be left until the end. Think whether you will include it in each class. The authors believe that, in order to use it effectively, women and partners need practice to learn the skill thoroughly. It is ideal to allow time in each session for this.

After learning the sequence and understanding the principles, it is necessary to try out the skill first on yourself. After that, it should be practised on one or two willing colleagues and friends who are not familiar with it.

You will need to consider how you intend to introduce relaxation to a group. Initially you could examine the causes and effects of stress with the women and their partners and exchange views on what stress-coping strategies they might use. This will also provoke discussion into the feelings of both partners. As a lead-in to teaching relaxation, the position of tension can be considered and actually felt by the group taking up a tense position.

The technique of choice should then be explained and the value of its use. Follow this by practice in a chosen position, repeating the sequence twice for the first few times. Progression is made during the weeks of practice by using less comfortable positions and a quicker, more active response in practice for labour along with breathing awareness. This will be the "ripple" relaxation where the sequence is run through quickly to gain a position of ease rapidly at the start of a contraction. At the end of the contraction, the ripple response is repeated.

The women (and partners) should always be told how long they will be relaxing if using the passive type. Usually, it will only be for a few minutes. (Refresher groups value this as time given to themselves and **this** baby and so enjoy longer relaxation).

Background music can be used as an aid to relaxation and noise and interruption should be kept to a minimum (especially at first). However, as relaxation is for "real life", the technique should gradually be used to switch off even from surrounding disturbance - after all, delivery suites are rarely totally quiet!

Remember that the woman will need time to adjust before gradually moving from relaxation. She should be encouraged to stretch slowly and perform some movements of the feet and hands to stimulate the circulation before sitting and standing.

Touch

Simple touch can be an excellent progression to use with couples or women working together in order to develop non-verbal communication based on touch *(Kitzinger, 1978)*. The partner learns to recognise areas of tension and the woman learns to respond to touch. Partners can place their hands gently but firmly on, for example, the shoulders in order to encourage low relaxation position. It offers women the chance to learn to relax while being touched which will be practice for labour. Touching is also contact and a reminder to the woman that she is not alone.

Massage

For thousands of years, massage or laying on of hands has been used to heal and soothe. It is another means of contact, giving reassurance, warmth, pleasure, comfort and renewed vitality. Massage involves systematic stroking, effleurage, kneading and/or pressure of the soft tissues. It relieves pain by stimulating the natural production of endorphins and encephalins, and may also trigger the pain-gate closing mechanism *(Wells, 1988)*. The techniques can be introduced in antenatal sessions for benefit during pregnancy, labour and general living.

Imagery and suggestion

Imagery and suggestion may be incorporated into other relaxation techniques. Concentration is on a mental image rather than on the physical state. To give the mind something happy and pleasant to think about, many suggestions are given, for example, a walk under trees, a garden or a favourite scene. Music, carefully chosen, may be played in the background. Each woman and partner must choose for themselves what image is right for them, as some may cause tension rather than aid relaxation; for example, using waves of the sea may cause tension if someone is frightened of water.

Hypnosis

Hypnosis is described as "an altered state of consciousness which is artificially induced and characterised by increased receptiveness to suggestions" *(Benson, 1988)*. It is capable of producing an anaesthetic effect, but it is used infrequently in labour as it is very time-consuming and is not successful for everyone.

Transcendental meditation (TSM)

Transcendental meditation is a simple skill involving the use of a mantra - secret word, sound or phrase - by the woman. This is repeated over and over again whilst resting in a comfortable position and a quiet environment. Practice is required at least twice a day. TSM has been shown to produce the relaxation response. The woman would be deeply relaxed but mentally active *(Benson, 1988)*.

Yoga

The technique of Yoga includes relaxation and breathing, and a woman who has used this method prior to pregnancy may choose to continue to practise it for childbirth. However as Yoga includes postures and stretching which may not be suitable for all pregnant women, the authors advise women not to take up this technique for the first time when they become pregnant. Yoga teachers may, however, be trained in holding classes just for women in pregnancy which will be especially adapted to avoid exercises which could be harmful at this time. As with all exercise sessions women must be advised to check that the teachers are fully qualified.

Relaxation techniques are coping skills for life which, once really learnt, are never forgotten. Although educators aim at their use in labour and delivery, they should also encourage their application in everyday living to deal with stressful situations.

References

Benson H. *The Relaxation Response*. Glasgow: Collins, 1988.

Health Education. *The New Pregnancy Book*. London: Health Education Authority, 1993.

Holmes T.H., Rahe R.H. The social readjustment rating scale. *J. Psychosom. Res*. 1967;11:213

Jacobsen E. *Progressive Relaxation*. Chicago: University of Chicago Press, 1938.

Kitzinger S. *The Experience of Childbirth*. 4th Edn. London: Pelican Books, 1978.

Madders J. *Stress and Relaxation*. London: Martin Dunnitz, 1979.

Mitchell L. *Simple Relaxation*. 2nd Edn. London: John Murray, 1987.

Wells P.E. Manipulative procedures. In: Wells P.E., Frampton V., Bowsher D., Eds. *Pain: Management and Control in Physiotherapy*. Oxford: Heinemann, 1988.

Woodrow Y. Relaxation Techniques in Prenatal Education. In: Wilder E., Ed. *Obstetric and Gynecologic Physical Therapy*. New York: Churchill Livingstone, 1988.

Further reading

Benson H. *The Relaxation Response*. Glasgow: Collins, 1988.

Madders J. *Stress and Relaxation*. London: Martin Dunnitz, 1979.

Mitchell L. *Simple Relaxation*. London: John Murray, 1987.

CHAPTER 5

Coping Strategies for Labour

One of the main reasons couples give for attending antenatal preparation classes is that they want to learn about labour and how to cope. To prepare couples for labour, we need to look at the problems they may face and suggest some coping strategies that they might consider.

Problems in labour:
- fear of the known or the unknown
- pain of contractions
- fear of being unable to cope
- tension
- hyperventilation

The authors found that the first three were the most common problems volunteered by couples, the others being the possible consequences of the failure to deal adequately with these three.

As antenatal educators our aims should be to:

- allay fear
- discuss relief of pain
- suggest coping strategies for use in labour
- teach relaxation techniques
- prevent hyperventilation

Discussion, visual aids and visits to the delivery suite will all help to allay fear and to reassure the couples. A session devoted to the methods of pain relief available in the unit will help them to make informed decisions when the time comes. Couples should be encouraged to discuss their care with their midwife and may wish to fill in a birth plan stating their preferences if all goes well.

Sessions during which coping strategies are practised will help the woman through the contractions and build up her confidence so that she will be able to cope with each contraction as it comes. If the woman is able to 'ride' her contractions, then tension and hyperventilation should be minimised or avoided.

Physical preparation for labour

The teaching of skills for labour has changed throughout the years with emphasis today being on a psychophysical approach which includes relaxation and breathing awareness. In the past, some suggested breathing techniques interfered with the natural rhythm of respiration and led to hyperventilation and subsequent criticism of the teachers. The commonly accepted way of dealing with this nowadays is to allow the woman to recognise and respond to the needs of her own body.

Teachers should revise their respiratory knowledge and the effects of various breathing techniques in labour.

Respiration in Labour

Respiration is controlled automatically by the respiratory centre in the brain which can be overridden by voluntary control. The respiratory centre responds to the level of carbon dioxide in the blood flowing through the centre. Any difference in this level of carbon dioxide will cause alterations in the rate or depth of respiration to normalise the level. Several factors cause the level to be altered, the commonest of which is exercise. Exercise uses energy and increases carbon dioxide output which automatically causes the respiratory centre to alter the rate or depth of respiration until the level is normal once more. A typical example of this is the way our breathing alters involuntarily when we run up a flight of steps.

Other factors affecting the respiratory centre are fear, apprehension, excitement, anger, frustration and pain. Most of these are exhibited in labour together with strong uterine contractions which use oxygen and produce excess carbon dioxide. If this occurs, the respiratory centre, which is more sensitive in pregnancy *(Metcalfe et al., 1988, Polden and Mantle, 1990)*, will automatically correct the situation. However, if the woman voluntarily superimposes deep or rapid breathing, she is in danger of causing the opposite situation, hyperoxygenation or too much oxygen. This is more commonly known as hyperventilation or overbreathing. The symptoms of this state are very unpleasant and frightening - dizziness, pallor, sweating, palpitations and tingling in the face and/or extremities. Hyperventilation occurred frequently when levels of breathing were practised as in psychoprophylaxis *(Buxton, 1965)*. Women should be aware of the possibility and dangers of hyperventilation and how to correct the situation, should it arise, by breathing into their own cupped hands to restore the carbon dioxide level quickly.

To avoid causing hyperventilation, antenatal teachers are now discouraging the practice of deep or rapid breathing patterns in labour and are instead, encouraging the mother to tune in to her own natural breathing rhythm and needs. This "tuning in" is often called "breathing awareness" and is a calm, regular breathing which reinforces relaxation as described in Chapter 4.

Of the two phases of respiration, expiration is the relaxing one. It is useful for women to concentrate on the outward breath and to practise tuning into the slight pause before inspiration follows. We always breathe in and no-one needs exhorting to do so, but on some occasions we need reminding to breathe out, or to do so more slowly. Breathing should never be a group activity where the members are instructed to 'breathe in and breathe out' in time with each other. Each person should be advised to breathe at his or her own individual rate and to think especially about the outward breath. It is suggested that a slow, deep breathing in labour gives better alveolar ventilation which increases the oxygen and decreases the carbon dioxide levels as necessary *(Stradling, 1984)*. This would be more beneficial than the rapid shallow breathing formerly suggested.

As described in Chapter 4, relaxation and respiration are very closely linked and to prevent hyperventilation in labour, practising the chosen relaxation technique in a comfortable and appropriate position will promote natural breathing awareness.

Chapter 9 contains instructions for a few carefully-chosen stretching exercises which women may like to practise in preparation for labour.

Comfortable positions for first stage labour

During the first stage, the labouring woman is trying to conserve her energy and allow the dilatation of the cervix to take place without attempting to resist the contractions. To achieve this, the couple will need to acquire some coping skills to help them through this long, tedious and often frustrating phase of labour. To facilitate relaxation in labour, the technique should be tried out in comfortable positions during pregnancy. Obviously no-one can predict what will be a comfortable position when labour is in progress, but the couple will have some alternatives to try.

If the contractions are felt mainly in the back, the woman may find a forward leaning position comfortable. For instance, sitting astride a chair, kneeling with arms supported or standing leaning forward against a wall or partner, all relieve the weight from the lumbar spine.

Many women are happier to be mobile during the first stage and some find relief with pelvic rocking and rhythmic pelvic gyrations during the contractions.

Fig. 5.1 *Alternative positions of ease for the first stage of labour*

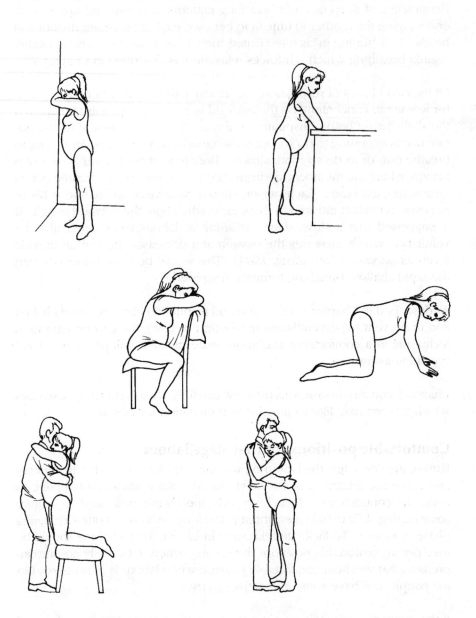

The physiological method of relaxation described in Chapter 4 is possible in any position. The joints, shoulders and fingers, can be checked quickly at the start of the contraction (ripple effect).

A general 'outline plan of action' for a contraction may be helpful for the couple to practise. If the woman understands the importance of relaxing through the contraction, she is much more likely to do so. A positive approach to each one will help the relaxation, whereas a negative one will encourage tension. So a woman could be advised to

- – greet the contraction positively
- – assume a comfortable position of ease
- – sigh out and check that her shoulders and hands are relaxed
- – tune in to her low, slow breathing throughout the contraction
- – give a sigh of relief at the end

This 5-point approach forms a helpful coping routine for labour which can be practised antenatally. The woman will need to concentrate on coping with the contractions and may need to be reminded not to try to hold a conversation at the same time! It will be necessary for her to check her relaxation at the end of each contraction and, if there is time, to use the passive technique between contractions.

The varied positions of ease shown in Fig. 5.1 should prove useful during the first stage of labour. The woman may need to change her position frequently depending on the distribution of pain and her choice of pain relief. Alteration of position during the first stage leads to productive uterine contractions *(Roberts et al., 1983)*. The emphasis nowadays is on keeping mobile, but there will be a time when the woman feels the need to adopt a resting position during the stronger contractions: rocking chairs, beanbags and a variety of arm chairs may be comfortable now.

S.O.S. breathing

If, as labour progresses, the woman finds herself breathing more quickly and beginning to tense during the contractions, concentrating more on the outward breath and audibly sighing out the air may help. This **S**ighing **O**ut **S**lowly breathing is often called **SOS** breathing and is used to prevent the emergency which could follow prolonged hyperventilation. Sighing out not only slows down the rate of breathing but also relaxes tense shoulders at the same time.

End of first stage

It may be useful to adapt the breathing slightly towards the end of the first stage of labour if there is a premature desire to push. The instinctive reaction is to take in a deep breath, hold it and bear down unless advised not to do so. Alteration of position is the most effective way of avoiding premature pushing and the woman can be helped into a side-lying position or, more effective still, a kneeling position with head resting on forearms. This will relieve the pressure from the anterior lip of the cervix.

Fig. 5.2 Knee chest position to avoid pushing

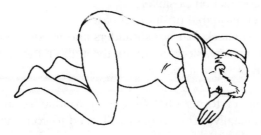

However, interrupted "breathing in threes" will also help to prevent pushing. This breathing adaptation is variously known as puff-puff-blow, pant-pant-blow or ooh-ooh-aah breathing and its aim is to prevent the diaphragm from fixing and increasing intra-abdominal pressure. (Panting, as used briefly for the crowning of baby's head, could cause hyperventilation if used during these long contractions). By giving 2 short blow-breaths out followed by a longer outward breath, the diaphragm is not allowed to fix, so pushing and hyperventilation are avoided. This type of breathing also requires increased concentration and may therefore be a diversionary technique. Some women may actually prefer to say "do-not-push", or count "one-two-three".

The woman will be emotionally and physically tired now and couples should be reminded of these aspects of the end of first stage, and partners warned that the mother-to-be may exhibit unusual behaviour and language at this time. This all helps to let off steam and aids relaxation but can be alarming for the labour companion if not prepared for it. The men can remind their partners that this emotional upset is very common at this time in labour and means that the second stage is about to commence.

Second stage of labour

Positions for the second stage of labour should be tried out in the antenatal classes. Squatting is an advantageous position for delivery as the pelvic outlet is 28% greater in area than in the supine position *(Russell, 1982)*. However not many women are able to squat comfortably, but need to discover this before deciding to give it a try in labour!

Gardosi designed a birthing cushion which allowed supported squatting and showed that there were shorter second stages and fewer forceps deliveries in the group that used this position *(Gardosi et al., 1989i)*. It has also been reported that kneeling, high sitting and standing postures also result in fewer forceps deliveries and less perineal trauma than a lying or semi-recumbent position *(Gardosi et al., 1989ii)*.

Fig. 5.3 Squatting for second stage of labour

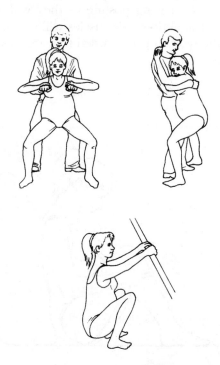

An alternative which is often more acceptable is kneeling on all fours or leaning over the back of the bed or with arms round partner's neck.

Fig. 5.4 Kneeling for second stage of labour

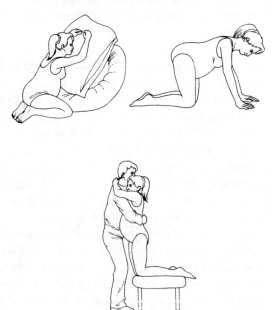

Many women are comfortable in a high sitting position but should not be allowed to slip down into a lying posture or they will then be pushing uphill against gravity. The abdominal muscles will not be able to work to their full potential if the woman is not curled forwards, as they will not be in their shortest position.

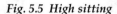

Fig. 5.5 High sitting

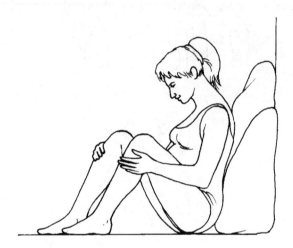

It is good to note that the practice of resting the mother's feet on the midwife's hips seems to have gone out of fashion. The extensor reflex pattern that this habit produced did not help the expulsive efforts and must have caused the midwife problems too!

Delivery positions for women with special needs may need to be discussed with an obstetric physiotherapist. For example, a woman who has presented with diastasis symphysis pubis antenatally should keep abduction of the hips to a minimum. Prone kneeling or side lying may be the better positions for her delivery *(Fry, 1992)*. The issue of "to push or not to push" must rest with the individual midwife and mother-to-be. The commonly taught method of pushing in the past was the use of the Valsalva manoeuvre, taking in a very deep breath, tucking the chin on the chest, closing the glottis and pushing for as long as possible. This was followed by a topping-up of breath and continued pushing for the duration of the contraction. The manoeuvre was so called after the physician of that name who used the procedure for expelling pus from the middle ear. In labour its use may lead to undesirable consequences, even loss of consciousness if maternal cerebral blood flow was already compromised *(Bush, 1992)*. It must be borne in mind that prolonged breath-holding followed by prolonged pushing using the Valsalva manoeuvre may be harmful to a baby who is already compromised because holding the breath for more than 6 seconds decreases the fetal circulation *(Caldeyro-Barcia, 1978)*. This prolonged pushing also puts additional strain on the fascia of the linea alba, rectus sheath and pelvic floor *(Noble, 1981)*; a perineum which has had time to thin out gradually is less likely to require an episiotomy *(Caldeyro-Barcia, 1979)*.

It seems, therefore, that it is better to discourage prolonged breath-holding and to encourage women to breathe out, then breathe in again in their own time. Bearing down should be encouraged only when there is the urge to do so and may be whilst the woman holds her breath (not for more than 6 seconds) or whilst she is breathing out. Several such bearing-down actions may be needed during the contraction. On some occasions, the midwife may need to coach the labouring woman in pushing, particularly if the uterine contractions cannot be felt, for example, following top up of epidural anaesthetic.

Between the contractions, the woman will benefit from quick total relaxation, which will allow her circulation and breathing to revert to normal before she begins the hard work of the next contraction. She may need reminding to relax her pelvic floor when she is aware of the pressure of the baby's head on the perineum. This will minimise the discomfort caused by the gradual stretching. The ultimate stretch experienced at the actual crowning can be simulated in the antenatal class to some extent by placing the little fingers in the corners of the mouth and pulling the lips sideways. The splitting/burning sensation is slightly similar to that felt in all diameters by those women who have not been given an episiotomy. The mouth seems to be empathetic with the pelvic floor and it is suggested that if the mouth is slack then the pelvic floor will also be relaxed *(Kitzinger, 1977)*.

Deep panting or 'breathing in threes' will prevent pushing at the crowning and at this stage is unlikely to cause ventilatory problems. The woman may need to be reminded to work with her midwife at this time and her partner can help by reinforcing instructions.

Role of the partner in labour

Partners can play a very important role in the birth of their baby but only if both parents-to-be wish it. Men should not be forced into a position where they are not totally happy because they feel it is expected of them. Neither should the woman feel that she must have a companion if she would rather not. Most delivery suites welcome a labour companion of either sex, but usually women in a stable relationship choose their partner. Apart from being a companion and an emotional and physical support, the partner can be responsible for various tasks whih will not only help the woman but will also assist the staff.

Ideally the couple will have attended at least one joint session on labour, better still a whole course, so the man can reinforce coping mechanisms learnt at the classes and remind his partner about her breathing and relaxation techniques. He may even breathe in time with her during the contractions and he is ideally placed to recognise if his partner starts to tense or panic-breathe. He can reinforce instructions from the midwifery staff and remind his partner of the milestones reached along the way. It is very comforting for the woman to have a close companion with whom she can completely relax and share her doubts and worries and enjoy the physical reassurance that close contact can bring. This contact may take the form of merely holding hands, stroking, brow-mopping or massage. The partner can be the one to help the woman into different positions as labour progresses and to support her in her chosen position during the second stage contractions. Between the contractions, he may find himself stretching or massaging her legs and feet as cramp is a common problem at this time. Finally, his presence and active support at the actual birth is the start of a new family life which both partners will share.

Teaching coping strategies

Teaching relaxation has been discussed in Chapter 4, but it might be helpful to hold a "rehearsal of labour" for couples and talk through imaginary contractions whilst they adopt any of the differnt positions that have been suggested. For example:

Early first stage

"You may feel the very early contractions as slight backache or period pains but they are more uncomfortable than painful. They may last up to 40 seconds and may be up to 30 minutes apart. If it is night-time try to rest, but during the day you may prefer to carry on with everyday activities, have a light snack, relax in a warm bath or pass the time watching television".

First stage contractions

"The contractions are now stronger and you may describe them as very uncomfortable or even painful. They may last 50 to 60 seconds and be 5 to 10 minutes apart. You may wish to remain active but concentrate on each contraction as it comes. Now is the time to put your 5-point plan into action:

- – greet the contraction positively and sigh out
- – check that you are in a comfortable position
- – check shoulders and hands are relaxed
- – breathe low and slow and concentrate on the outward breath. As the contraction rises to a peak, continue to breathe easily throughout
- – give a sigh of relief at the end as the contraction dies away, and check you are relaxed".

Later first stage contractions

"By now the contractions will be very strong, may last about 60 seconds and be only 2 to 3 minutes apart. You may have had some form of pain relief and prefer to be less active. The contraction will be at its peak for about 45 seconds and you will feel as though it is taking over your whole body - let it, don't try to resist or fight it. Your 5-point plan still holds good but you may need to concentrate on **S**ighing **O**ut **S**lowly during the contraction - your partner can do it with you. Stay relaxed and don't forget the long sigh at the end".

End of first stage

"This is a transitional stage before the uterus starts to push the baby down the birth canal. The contractions now are very powerful and long and may be every 2 minutes. You may feel or be sick and there may be pressure on your back passage which makes you want to push at the peak of the contraction. **Never push** until your midwife has confirmed that you are in the second stage, instead roll onto your side or into the kneeling position with your head on your forearms. This is where the "breathing in threes" technique should help you through the contraction. At the end of this one you deserve 2 sighs of relief!

You have been working very hard and will feel emotionally and physically drained. You may think that you cannot carry on any longer, you may even turn on your partner and tell him to go. These are recognisable reactions at this time and mean that there is not much longer to go before you are in the second stage".

Second stage contractions

"Sometimes the contractions diminish for a short time after full dilatation of the cervix. You can make the most of this short rest by relaxing. When the contractions return you will probably feel as though you want to bear down with them, but there is no need to push unless you have the urge to do so. When you are pushing, adopt your chosen position and bear down steadily, remembering not to hold your breath for more than 6 seconds. You may need 4 or 5 pushes with each contraction. Relax completely between contractions and breathe slowly and deeply. Gradually you will feel the pressure of your baby's head stretching your perineum; this is when you need to relax your pelvic floor during the contractions".

Crowning

"As the baby's head is stretching the perineum to its limit, you will feel a tight, burning sensation. Stay calm and listen to your midwife. She will tell you to stop pushing and to pant deeply just for a few seconds, then to push, perhaps to pant again and then push again. This will allow your baby's head to be born slowly. During the next contraction you may be asked to pant again as the shoulders are delivered, the rest of the baby will slide out easily.

At last the hard work is over - Congratulations!"

References

Bush A. Cardiopulmonary effects of pregnancy and labour. *Journal of the Association of Chartered Physiotherapists in Obstetrics and Gynaecology.* 1992;71:3

Buxton R., St.J. Breathing in labour: the influence of psychoprophylaxis. *Nursing Mirror.* 1965;viii

Caldeyro-Barcia R. The influence of maternal position on labour and the influence of maternal bearing-down efforts in the second stage of labour on fetal well-being. In: Simpkin P. and Reinke, Eds. *Kaleidescope of Childbearing Preparation, Birth and Nurturing.* Seattle: Pennypress, 1978.

Caldeyro-Barcia R. Physiological and psychological bases for the modern and humanised management of normal labour. In: *Recent Progress in Perinatal Medicine and Prevention of Congenital Anomaly.* Tokyo:Ministry of Health and Welfare. 1979;77

Fry D. Diastasis symphysis pubis. *Journal of the Association of Chartered Physiotherapists in Obstetrics and Gynaecology.* 1992;71:10

Gardosi J., Hutson N., B-Lynch C. Randomised controlled trial of squatting in the second stage of labour. *Lancet.* 1989(i);ii:74

Gardosi J., Sylvester S., B-Lynch C. Alternative positions in the second stage of labour: a randomised controllled trial. *Brit. J. Obstet. Gynaec.* 1989(ii);96:1290

Kitzinger S. *Education and Counselling for Childbirth.* London: Ballière Tindall, 1977.

Metcalfe J., Stocks M.K., Barron D.H. Maternal physiology during gestation. In: Knobil E & Neill J. Eds. *The Physiology of Reproduction.* New York: Raven Press, 1988.

Noble E. Controversies in maternal effort during labour and delivery. *J. Nurse-Midwifery.* 1981;26:13

Polden M., Mantle J. *Physiotherapy in Obstetrics and Gynaecology.* London: Butterworth Heinemann, 1990.

Roberts J.E., Mendez-Bauer C., Wodell D.A. The effects of maternal position on uterine contractility and efficiency. *Birth.* 1983;10:243

Russell J.G.B. The rationale of primitive delivery positions. *Brit. J. Obstet. Gynaec.* 1982;89:712

Stradling J. Respiratory physiology during labour. *Midwife, Health Visitor and Community Nurse.* 1984;20:38

CHAPTER 6

Transcutaneous Electrical Nerve Stimulation (TENS)

Transcutaneous electrical nerve stimulation (TENS, TES or TNS), has been used as a method of pain relief for many years and is widely used today, particularly for chronic pain and that associated with terminal illness. However, it is only relatively recently that it has been used for more acute pain and found to be of advantage *(Woolf, 1989)*. In 1983 Spembley manufactured a TENS unit especially designed for use in labour. This was the first unit of its type in the UK and is called the Obstetric Pulsar. Since then, other manufacturers have competed for the market by adapting existing models with varying degrees of success.

TENS is a low-frequency current applied to the skin via pairs of electrodes. These can be placed over the painful area or over the nerve routes supplying the area of pain. The current produces a tingling sensation, the intensity (strength) of which can be altered by the individual. The pulsed low-frequency modality encourages the release of cerebrospinal endogenous opiates (endorphins) which are the body's own natural pain-relieving agents and these raise the individual's pain threshold *(Thompson, 1989)*. The obstetric model differs in that it has a high-frequency modality which, when activated, brings in a continuous high-frequency current to boost the low-frequency current to give added pain relief. It is thought that this higher frequency current works on the pain-gate theory and lessens the pain impulses received by the brain *(Wall, 1985)*. The high-frequency modality is brought into play by pressing a patient-demand switch and stopped by pressing it once more.

Electrodes

For labour, 4 electrodes which are of sufficient length to cover the nerve roots supplying the uterus and cervix (T10 - L1) and the birth canal and pelvic floor (S2 - S4) are required. The recommended size of the electrodes is 10cm x 4cm, and they can be of different materials. The original and most economical electrodes are made of carbon-impregnated rubber which need a coupling medium of gel under the complete surface to ensure continuous contact with the skin. More recently, disposable electrodes have been introduced which are applied to a wet skin and are self-adherent. A third type (supplied with hire units) has a very sticky self-adhesive surface and in theory can be re-used a few times, but in practice this is not recommended for reasons of hygiene and because the electrodes become less adhesive.

Fig. 6.1 TENS unit

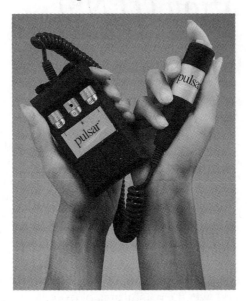

Use of TENS

TENS works best for women who apply it early in labour as it takes about 40 minutes for the endorphins to be maximally released *(Salar et al., 1981)*. It can help the woman to cope in the early latent phase before labour is fully established. It has been shown that the levels of pain and distress-related thoughts experienced during the latent phase of labour were predictive of the length of labour and obstetric outcomes *(Wuitchik et al., 1989)*.

When the woman feels in need of further pain relief, she can activate the high-frequency mode at the start of the contraction and use for the duration of the contraction, returning to the low-frequency mode at the end.

There are no side effects from TENS and no depression of respiration *(Woolf, 1989)*, a pacemaker in situ being the only contraindication to its use. It is a safe non-invasive therapy which, if required, can be used in conjunction with other forms of pain relief as labour progresses. TENS does not give a pain-free labour and this fact must be stressed to the woman and her partner. However, for the woman who wishes to be in control of her pain relief it is a useful addition to other available analgesia. The general feeling among midwives is that TENS users who choose to have additional analgesia require lower doses than those who are not using TENS. However, this has never been documented, and would be difficult to establish.

Transcutaneous nerve stimulation can be used during suturing and to relieve afterpains as well as during labour itself.

Ideally women and their partners should be introduced to the TENS unit during the antenatal classes. Then, if they are interested in trying or applying it, a group or individual session can be arranged where the women can experience its sensation on their backs and their partners practise siting the electrodes (see Ch. 10). The sensation on the back is usually preferred to that on the forearm and women need to feel it before going to the expense of hiring a unit.

Siting the electrodes

The woman should sit on the edge of the bed whilst her partner stands behind on the other side of the bed. She should have her arms relaxed by her side and her back exposed down to the gluteal cleft. The area from the level of the bra strap down to the gluteal cleft should be washed and dried to remove any natural skin grease which could impede the electrical current. The electrodes are attached to the leads making sure no metal is exposed. To site the upper 2 electrodes, T10 is palpated. The easiest way of locating this is to feel for the inferior angle of the scapula with the little fingers of each hand, then reach across to the spine at the *same level* with the thumbs. The vertebra palpated will be T 7, count 3 vertebrae down to find T10. (A good guide is the lower border of the bra strap in most women). The upper borders of one set of electrodes should be fixed at the level of T10 about 2cm either side of the thoracic spine (approx 5 cm apart), with the leads hanging downwards (see Fig. 6.2). If the reusable carbon electrodes are being used, they should be thoroughly covered with the conducting gel supplied and held in place with a piece of Mefix large enough to cover both electrodes. The top of the second pair of electrodes is placed at the level of the sacral dimples (S2) with the lower borders reaching down to just above the gluteal cleft. The leads should point upwards.

The electrodes should not be placed on the abdomen as there may be a slight chance of interference on the fetal monitor if a scalp electrode is in use. It has been reported that interference has been noted occasionally when both electrodes are placed dorsally, but this has been with older monitors and disappears when the intensity of the TENS is reduced.With both sets of electrodes in place and checked and the unit switched off, the plug end of each lead is inserted into the sockets on the top of the TENS unit. The woman should know which electrodes are attached to which control so she can increase the intensity of each channel independently. A much better effect is achieved if the woman is in complete control of the unit from the start. Once the electrodes are in place the stimulator can be clipped on to her clothes and she can remain active or adopt any position she wishes.

Fig. 6.2 Position of TENS electrodes for pain relief in labour

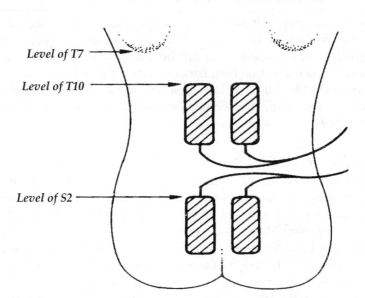

The intensity (strength) of the 2 channels can be increased as required using the relevant intensity control (see Fig. 6.1). The frequency of the pulses, which is a personal choice, can also be varied by altering the rate control (see Fig. 6.1). This does not affect the intensity of the output, only the rate of the pulses. The manufacturers of the Spembley Pulsar unit advise an initial frequency of 7 on the dial, then further adjustment to meet the personal needs of each individual. However, some TENS units have a pre-set, unalterable frequency.

Unless a delivery suite has sufficient units to allow women to take one home just prior to their expected delivery date, hiring their own is often preferred. The hired units will include the easy-to-apply self-adhesive electrodes which do not require gel. There will be 2 pairs for use in labour and generally, depending on the company, an additional pair for practice in the 2 weeks prior to birth. It is inadvisable to try out the procedure before 38 weeks of pregnancy (see the manufacturer's guide). Hire contracts are usually for 4 weeks starting at 38 weeks with an additional fee if the unit is not returned after this time.

Fig. 6.3 A TENS hire package

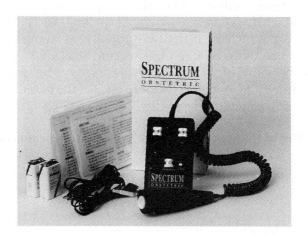

Criteria for selection of a TENS unit

Midwives and health visitors should be aware of the different models on the market before giving out literature to couples. The cheapest deal is not necessarily the best option. Crothers (1992) tried out 2 different units during her own labour and decided that certain criteria were important.

She was a member of the working party of The Association of Chartered Physiotherapists in Obstetrics & Gynaecology who devised the following criteria for the suitability of TENS equipment for use in labour:

- sufficient intensity/amplitude to relieve pain.
- scope to alter the frequency.
- both pulsed and continuous mode.
- additional amplitude with continuous mode.
- simple and easy to apply and operate.
- correct instructions for placing the electrodes.
- press/release booster button, not press/hold.
- electrodes to measure a minimum of 10cm x 4cm.
- separate intensity control for each pair of electrodes.
- durable electrodes, leads and attachments.
- transmission gel must be suitable for adequate conduction with carbon electrodes.

Some delivery suites hire out their own units, but this can be an onerous undertaking. A new battery and electrodes are needed for each user and the unit should be checked after its return to the labour suite before being re-issued.

TENS for post-caesarean delivery

Following caesarean section, where the mother is not offered self-administered pain relief via Cardiff pump or an epidural, TENS may be used for post-operative pain relief. It has been found that women who used TENS after caesarean births required less narcotic analgesia and so were better able to cope with their babies *(Hollinger, 1986)*. The electrodes are usually placed above a Pfannenstiel incision towards the outer sides of the abdomen as this is where most pain is felt.

Fig. 6.4 Position of TENS electrodes for relief of post caesarean wound pain

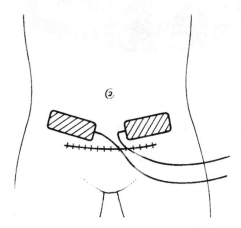

One set of electrodes only may be applied, or a second pair may be placed either side of the first and second lumbar vertebrae. The low-frequency mode is all that is necessary at rest, but, if the mother needs to cough or move about, the high-frequency can be used as during contractions.

The UKCC's latest advice with regard to midwives using TENS is contained in the following Registrar's Letter 8/1991:

The Council has accepted the recommendation of its Midwifery Committee that midwives may, on their own responsibility, manage pain relief in labour by the use of transcutaneous nerve stimulation (TNS) **provided that:**

1. they have received adequate and appropriate <u>instruction</u>*, which is a matter to be determined by agreed local policy and*

2. <u>safety standards</u> *conform to those laid down by the Department of Health Medical Devices Directorate in England, or equivalent body in Scotland, Wales or Northern Ireland. The current standard for all medical equipment is set out in British Standard specification BS 5724 Part 1 1989.*

References

Crothers E. TENS in labour. *Journal of the Association of Chartered Physiotherapists in Obstetrics and Gynaecology.* 1992;70:26

Hollinger J.L. Transcutaneous electric nerve stimulation after caesarean birth. *Physical Therapy.* 1986;66:36

Salar G, Job I, Mingrino S, Bosio A, & Trabucchi M. Effect of transcutaneous electrotherapy on CSF beta endorphin content in patients without pain problems. *Pain.* 1981;10:169

Thompson J.W. Pharmacology of Transcutaneous Electrical Nerve Stimulation (TENS). *Journal of the Intractable Pain Society of Great Britain and Ireland.* 1989;7:33

Wall P.D. The discovery of transcutaneous electrical nerve stimulation. *Physiotherapy.* 1985; 71:348

Woolf C.J. Transcutaneous and implanted nerve stimulation. In: Wall P.D. and Melzack R, Eds. *Textbook of Pain.* Edinburgh: Churchill Livingstone, 1989.

Wuitchik M., Bakal D., Lipshitz J. The clinical significance of pain and cognitive activity in latent labour. *Obst. Gynec.* 1989;73:35

Further Reading

Wall P.D., Melzack R., Eds. *Textbook of Pain.* Edinburgh: Churchill Livingstone, 1989.

CHAPTER 7

Physiological Changes and Physical Problems in the Puerperium

Most physiological changes which occurred during pregnancy gradually resolve during the 6-8 weeks following delivery, so that at the end of the puerperium the mother should be back to her pre-pregnancy state. Some systems revert more quickly than others. The musculoskeletal system can still manifest some effects as long as 6 months postpartum *(Polden and Mantle, 1990)*, which has a bearing on the exercises and advice that should be given to women at this time.

The main physiological changes occurring in the puerperium are:

–   involution of the uterus which starts immediately following delivery and should be complete after 6 weeks.
–   lactation which occurs as a result of the action of prolactin initially secreted by the anterior pituitary gland.
–   physiological changes in other body systems which return the body to its pre-pregnancy state.

The important ones to note here, because of their effect on the physical rehabilitation of the postnatal mother, are:

Cardiovascular

Smooth muscle tone in the walls of the veins begins to improve, blood volume decreases, the viscosity of the blood returns to normal and cardiac output and blood pressure drop to their pre-pregnant levels. There may be some residual oedema in the feet and hands from pregnancy, from increased fluid input in labour, from congestion due to prolonged pushing in the second stage or from relative immobility immediately postpartum.

Musculoskeletal

The effects of relaxin and progesterone (see Ch. 2) on the fibrous tissue, muscles and ligaments ceases, but it may take 4-5 months *(Calguneri et al., 1982)* for these to be reversed. However it has been suggested that it can take up to 6 months before joint laxity regresses to near its pre-pregnancy state *(Polden and Mantle, (1990)*. An increased kyphosis and lordosis in pregnancy may persist for up to 12 weeks postnatally *(Bullock, 1991)*. In the immediate postpartum period, the ligaments are at their longest and the joints are at their least stable.

The abdominal and pelvic-floor muscles are stretched and weak. The length of the abdominals increases by approximately two thirds in a primigravid woman with an average weight gain. In a multiparous woman this length may even double by term *(Polden, 1985)*. There could also be diastasis of the rectus abdominis muscles due to the hormonal effect on the linea alba coupled with the increasing bulk of the uterus. Persistent use of the Valsalva manoeuvre during the second stage of labour (see Ch. 5) increases the stress on the abdominal muscles and may be a contributary factor to diastasis *(Noble, 1988)*.

The pelvic-floor muscles have supported the weight of the uterus and contents during pregnancy and have stretched during delivery. The composition of the fascial layer of the pelvic floor has altered due to the hormonal influence of relaxin and has been strained by the increased weight of the pelvic contents during pregnancy (see Ch. 2). It too will have stretched at delivery and will take time to resume its pre-pregnant form. The perineum may have been torn or cut and repaired and may be bruised, swollen and sore. It is possible that there could be some degree of urinary incontinence in the early puerperium. It has been suggested that some women lose control over their pelvic floor muscles following intense postpartum perineal pain *(Shepherd, 1980)*.

Respiratory

There is no further mechanical blocking of full descent of the diaphragm or full ventilation of the lower lungs by the uterus. The mother is now able to expand the whole of her lungs and should be encouraged to do so.

Rehabilitation of the stretched musculature and advice on back care and increasing activities is described in Chapter 8. Diligent practice of postnatal exercises should hasten the postnatal recovery and avoid problems which might otherwise occur. However mothers do often suffer from complications after delivery, some of which may become long-term.

SOME PHYSICAL POSTNATAL PROBLEMS

A bruised and oedematous perineum

This can be extremely painful and incapacitating for the new mother. Advice about positions for feeding may help the mother's comfort; sitting with a pillow under each ischial tuberosity to relieve the pressure on the perineum or side-lying with a pillow between the knees. As rubber rings are frowned upon in many establishments, specially constructed inflatable cushions are being tested. These cushions can be inflated to suit individual comfort and appear to have all the advantages of the rubber ring without the disadvantages. A very comfortable resting position is prone-lying with a pillow under the hips and another under the head and shoulders. Many mothers forget that they can lie on their tummies once more!

The pain can be eased considerably by the application of ice which is cheap, readily available and easy to apply. It may be flaked or crushed and placed inside a polythene bag or gauze which is covered with a clean, disposable cloth and placed on the painful area for no longer than 5-10 minutes. If the mother is applying ice to her own perineum she should be reminded of the risks of a burn if the ice remains in contact with the skin. However, the painful area can be massaged for 5-10 minutes by an ice cube held in a disposable cloth. Ice should not be used for longer than the advised length of time and should be crushed if in continuous contact to avoid the possibility of ice burns. The pain relieving properties of ice for recent injuries has been consistently documented *(Palastanga, 1988, Knight, 1989, Moore and James, 1989)*. The latter compared the application of Epifoam, Hamamelis water and ice. Each gave good pain relief to two thirds of the women on the first day, but ice gave better pain relief on subsequent days. The most comfortable position for the mother is usually side-lying on an inco-pad, with a pillow between her knees. Much discussion has taken place about the use of ice delaying healing *(Grant et al., 1989)*, but the authors consider that ice, if applied correctly, is a valid treatment for the painful perineum as the initial vasoconstriction is followed by a vasodilatation which will increase circulation and promote healing *(Palastanga, 1988)*.

An obstetric physiotherapist will be able to treat the perineum with therapeutic ultrasound or pulsed electromagnetic energy (PEME). The latter is sometimes called pulsed shortwave, although this term is not technically correct, and is very often referred to as *Megapulse* which is actually the trade name for one particular model. Both therapeutic ultrasound and pulsed electromagnetic energy have similar physiological effects, relieving pain and reducing oedema, but there is no evidence that the rate of healing is speeded up by treatment with either modality *(Grant et al., 1989)*. Pelvic floor exercises in themselves help to relieve the pressure on the perineum especially in standing or sitting. The rhythmical contraction and relaxation of the muscles helps to improve the local circulation and remove waste products from the area.

Gentle warmth from an infra-red heat lamp or reading lamp at home may help to ease the pain as may warm, but not hot, baths.

Haematoma

Haematomata of the rectus sheath or perineum respond very favourably to the application of therapeutic ultrasound or pulsed electro magnetic energy administered by the obstetric physiotherapist.

Haemorrhoids

Haemorrhoids can also be helped by the application of therapeutic ultrasound or pulsed electro -magnetic energy. The haemorrhoids are visibly reduced in size in a short space of time and the accompanying pain alleviated.

Diastasis recti

This is a condition where a gap of 3cm (2 fingers) or more appears between the 2 rectus muscles. It can occur towards the end of pregnancy when it is difficult to detect, or may occur during labour especially if there has been prolonged breath-holding with pushing during the second stage *(Noble, 1988)*. It is more common with multiple pregnancies, large babies and polyhydramnios, but may appear for seemingly no apparent reason in slim, fit women. It is thought that this might be due to inappropriate exercising during later pregnancy. In severe cases where the gap may be as much as 10cms, or even more, the mother may complain of constant backache as the abdominal muscles are no longer supporting the spine or pelvis. It can be a frightening condition for a mother as the intestines may be visible and she may feel that they may protrude even further on standing. It is easy to detect a severe diastasis from the visible 'peaking' of the recti on sitting up from the supine position, but each mother should be examined individually. Testing for diastasis recti is covered in detail in Chapter 8.

If a gap of 3cm (2 fingers) or more is palpated, size "J" or "K" tubigrip worn round the trunk from the xiphisternum to below the buttocks will give some support for the first few days. In extreme cases the tubigrip can be double thickness. Advice about posture, getting out of bed and special exercises for the rectus muscles are all important (see below), and, if available, an obstetric physiotherapist should be consulted. These women must be followed up and may require postnatal rehabilitation as out-patients. Support for the abdominals in subsequent pregnancies is advised as the diastasis can recur.

Fig. 7.1 Diastasis of recti postpartum

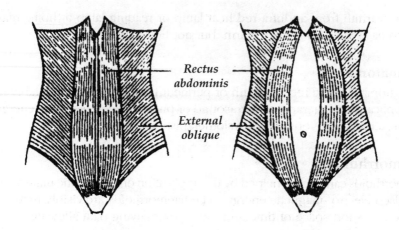

Rectus
abdominis

External
oblique

Special exercises for diastasis recti

If diastasis of 3cm (2 fingers) or more has been confirmed, the practice of strong exercises for the straight abdominals or any rotation exercises may increase the gap (see Ch. 8). Special attention should be paid to bringing the recti closer together and closing the gap by working the muscles in a straight direction only. The easiest exercise and one which can be performed in any position is **abdominal retraction.** The mother is taught to pull in the abdominal muscles, hold them tight for a count of 4, then slowly relax. **Pelvic tilting with head-lifting** exercises can be done in back-lying with the knees bent up and the feet flat on the bed.

Fig. 7.2 Pelvic tilting with head-lifting for diastasis recti

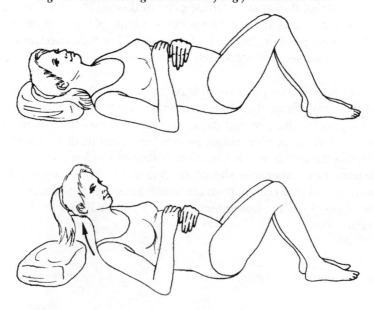

At first there should be 2 pillows supporting the head and shoulders and the mother's hands should be crossed over the abdomen. As she tightens the abdominals, tilts the pelvis and lifts the head slowly from the pillows, she is instructed to pull the opposing rectus muscles towards each other with her hands, breathing out gently as she does so. This position is held for a count of 4, before lowering the head down slowly.

As the gap closes, head and shoulder lifting can be added to the pelvic tilting, but if the recti start to peak, the head and shoulders must not be lifted further. **NB** The abdominals must always be tightened before head lifting takes place. Progressive exercises to be practised when the diastasis is less than 3cm (2 fingers) are described in Chapter 8.

DOUBLE-LEG RAISING AND SIT-UPS WITH STRAIGHT LEGS SHOULD NEVER BE PERFORMED.

Diastasis symphysis pubis

This condition may present in late pregnancy due to hormonal influence, or may occur as a result of the trauma of a difficult labour. Occasionally, however, the onset of symptoms can be 24-48 hours after delivery *(Fry, 1992)*, and is thought to be caused by swelling and increased pressure within the confines of the joint. This was first reported on in Malawi *(Driessen, 1987)*.

Complete separation requires bed rest and a trochanteric belt in the acute stage until the severe pain has subsided. The mother should be taught how to move in bed by keeping her knees bent and close together. As the pain subsides, the mother can be gently mobilised taking short steps with the aid of a walking frame or crutches. Some mothers have found it more comfortable to walk backwards, but they should be resting, not walking at all, if this is the case. Local pain relief can be given whilst the mother is on bed rest and might include therapeutic ultrasound or TENS administered by an obstetric physiotherapist. Ice could also be applied as described above in the treatment of the bruised perineum. Circulatory exercises should be stressed whilst the mother is immobile and abdominal retractions and pelvic tilting (see Ch. 8) may be commenced.

Backache

In the early postnatal period, backache is usually postural, unless the woman was troubled with joint or ligament problems during her pregnancy. If she chose epidural anaesthesia for labour, the woman may have adopted a poor back position without realising it. Advice on posture and positions, how to get in and out of bed and lifting are all necessary. Pelvic tilting exercises should ease the backache. Local heat from a warm bath, heat lamp (or hot water bottle wrapped in towels if at home) may give comfort. Very weak abdominals or a significant diastasis of recti will lead to an alteration in posture and low back pain *(Boissonnault and Kotarinos, 1988)*. It is thought that there could be a connection between long-term backache and epidural anaesthesia in labour *(MacArthur et al., 1990)*. More recent work now suggests that the backache is postural and not severe *(Russell et al., 1993)*.

Coccydynia

Coccydynia may be related to a previous injury, but is more usually caused by a difficult delivery. The pain may result from a bruised or displaced coccyx or rarely from a fracture *(Brunskill and Swain, 1987)*. It is a very painful condition which can incapacitate the mother and alternative positions for feeding etc. must be suggested. Many mothers find prone-lying on a pillow is a comfortable resting position. If the mother wants to sit, pillows can be arranged so there is no pressure on the coccyx, and an upright position will be the most comfortable. An inflatable cushion (see page 74) can be adjusted to give minimal pressure on the area and can be hired for use at home. Pain relief will almost definitely be required. An obstetric physiotherapist can apply therapeutic ultrasound or pulsed electromagnetic energy (see page 74) or interferential therapy for pain relief. This latter is a further electrotherapy modality which can be successful in relieving pain. It has been suggested that gentle mobilisations may also be helpful, and that TENS can be a valuable means of analgesia *(Polden and Mantle, 1990)*.

Urinary problems

Following delivery there is a physiological diuresis due to reduction in blood volume and increase in waste products. Some mothers, especially after an instrumental delivery, find it difficult to initiate micturition. They may be helped by performing regular pelvic-floor contractions in a warm bath. Alternatively, the mother may find that she is having difficulty in holding her urine long enough to get to the toilet and again pelvic-floor exercises should help these early problems.

Many women find that they leak a little urine when they cough, laugh, sneeze, lift objects or perform sudden movements. This symptom, known as **stress incontinence**, is common in pregnancy due to the hormonal influence on the pelvic floor plus the extra weight it is having to support (see Ch. 2). Sadly, it is thought that as many as 1 in 3 of all women who have had children suffer from this condition to a greater or lesser degree postnatally. In a study in 1990, it was found that 80% of primiparous women who had undergone vaginal deliveries showed electromyographic evidence of re-innervation of the pelvic-floor muscles 8 weeks postpartum *(Allen et al., 1990)*, showing that some denervation had taken place.

Most cases of stress incontinence will respond to an individually-designed course of pelvic-floor exercises and all mothers who have symptoms which persist after 12 weeks must be encouraged to get a referral to an obstetric physiotherapist either through their general practitioner or consultant.

Other common problems which may manifest themselves postnatally are **frequency, urgency and prolapse**. Following assessment, these conditions can respond favourably to an individual regime of bladder training, pelvic-floor exercises and electrotherapy. Midwives should avoid the practice of running taps to encourage micturition after delivery, as the authors know of a case where this practice initiated a long-term inappropriate response to running water.

Bowel problems

Fortunately faecal incontinence is much less common than urinary incontinence postnatally, but when present is an extremely distressing and embarrassing problem. It may be due to tearing or stretching of the anal sphincter or actual damage to the nerve supply to the pelvic-floor muscles *(Snooks et al., 1985)*. Depending on the severity of the nerve damage, function may not be restored for some weeks or in some cases it may be permanently impaired. All women complaining of faecal incontinence should be referred for specialist help from an obstetric physiotherapist.

Dyspareunia

Painful intercourse can be a most distressing side effect of labour. It is more common in women who have had episiotomies *(Kitzinger and Walters, 1981)* and may resolve over the following few weeks or last much longer. It has been stated that 23% of women report pain during intercourse as long as 3 months after delivery *(Sleep et al., 1984)*. If after trying alternative positions and the use of lubricants, the condition persists, the woman should be referred for physiotherapy treatment. McIntosh (1988) found that of 22 women who complained of dyspareunia at 3 months postpartum, only 5 did not experience any relief of symptoms after 12 treatments of therapeutic ultrasound. It has been suggested that some relief may be gained from the counselling and reassurance that accompanies the treatment of dyspareunia since women receiving placebo treatment improved *(Everett et al. ,1992)*.

References

Allen R.E., Hosker G.L., Smith A.R.B., Warrell D.W. Pelvic floor damage and childbirth: a neurophysiological study. *Brit. J. Obstet. Gynaec.* 1990;97:770

Boissonnault J.S., Kotarinos R.K. In: Wilder E. Ed. *Obstetric and Gynecologic Physical Therapy.* Edinburgh: Churchill Livingstone, 1988.

Brunskill P.J., Swain J.W. Spontaneous fracture of the coccygeal body during the second stage of labour. *J. Obstet. Gynaecol.* 1987;7:270

Bullock J.E. Changes in posture associated with pregnancy and the early postnatal period measured in standing. *Physiotherapy Theory and Practice*. 1991;7:103

Calguneri M., Bird H.A., Wright V. Changes in joint laxity occurring during pregnancy. *Ann. Rheum. Dis*. 1982;41:126

Driessen F. Postpartum pelvic arthropathy with unusual features. *Brit. J. Obstet. Gynaec*. 1987;94:870

Everett T., McIntosh J., Grant A. Ultrasound therapy for persistent postnatal perineal pain and dyspareunia - A randomised placebo-controlled trial. *Physiotherapy*. 1992;78:263

Fry D. Diastasis symphysis pubis. *Journal of the Association of Chartered Physiotherapists in Obstetrics and Gynaecology*. 1992;71:10

Grant A., Sleep J., McIntosh J., Ashurst H. Ultrasound and pulsed electromagnetic energy treatment for perineal trauma. A randomised placebo-controlled trial. *Brit. J. Obstet. Gynaec*. 1989;96:434

Kitzinger S., Walters R. *Some Women's Experience of Episiotomy*. London: National Childbirth Trust. 1981.

Knight K.L. Cryotherapy in sports injury management. In: Grisogono V. Ed. *Sports Injuries*, Edinburgh: Churchill Livingstone, 1989.

MacArthur C., Lewis W., Knox E.G., et al. Epidural anaesthesia and longterm backache after childbirth. *Br. Med. J*. 1990;301:9

McIntosh J. Research in Reading into treatment of perineal trauma and late dyspareunia. *Journal of the Association of Chartered Physiotherapists in Obstetrics and Gynaecology*. 1988;62:17

Moore W., James D.K. A random trial of three topical analgesic agents in the treatment of episiotomy pain following instrumental vaginal delivery. *J. Obstet. Gynaecol*. 1989;10:35

Noble E. *Essential Exercises for the Childbearing Year*, 3rd Edn. Boston: Houghton Mifflin, 1988.

Palastanga N.P. Heat and Cold. In: Wells P.E., Frampton V., Bowsher D. Eds. *Pain: Management and Control in Physiotherapy*. Oxford: Heinemann, 1988.

Polden M. Teaching postnatal exercises. *Midwives Chronicle & Nursing Notes*. 1985;10:271

Polden M. Mantle J. *Physiotherapy in Obstetrics and Gynaecology*. London: Butterworth-Heinemann, 1990.

Russell R., Groves P., Taub., O'Dowd J., Reynolds F. Assessing long term backache after childbirth. *Br. Med. J*. 1993;306:1299

Shepherd A. Re-education of the muscles of the pelvic floor. In: Mandelstam D. Ed. *Incontinence and its Management*. London: Croom Helm, 1980.

Sleep J.M., Grant A., Garcia J., Elbourne D., Spencer J.A.D., Chalmers I. West Berkshire perineal management trial. *Br. Med. J*. 1984;289:587

Snooks S.J., Swash M., Henry M.M. Setchell M. Risk factors in childbirth causing damage to the pelvic floor innervation. *Br. J. Surg*. 1985;72:Suppl.5,15

CHAPTER 8

Postnatal Exercises and Advice

Following delivery, the new mother's body begins its recovery and gradually returns to the pre-pregnancy state. Some rest and postnatal exercise will help this physiological process to take place smoothly. It is of great advantage if the mother has had opportunity to consider postnatal exercises prior to delivery. Although she may be suffering from fatigue, discomfort and the responsibilities of mothering, the subject should be broached with enthusiasm and the following simple exercises encouraged.

POSTNATAL EXERCISES FOLLOWING NORMAL DELIVERY

Circulatory exercises

These exercises should be performed as often as possible after delivery. They are intended to maintain and/or improve the mother's circulation in the immediate post-partum period when she could be at risk of deep venous thrombosis or other circulatory complications. The exercises may be done under or on top of the bedclothes several times every waking hour and should be continued until the mother is fully mobile and there is no oedema present. They are especially relevant after an epidural anaesthesia when there may be considerable oedema of feet and ankles.

Foot exercises

Sit or lie with the knees straight. Bend and stretch the ankles briskly at least 10 times, emphasising dorsiflexion rather than plantarflexion to avoid cramp. Keeping the knees and hips still, circle both ankles in as big a circle as possible at least 10 times in each direction.

Leg tightening

Sit or lie with the legs straight. Pull both feet upwards at the ankle and press the back of the knees down onto the bed. Hold this position for a count of 4, breathing normally, then relax. Repeat 5 times.

Fig. 8.1 Foot exercises

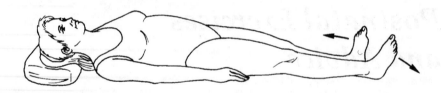

Deep breathing

Previous advice given antenatally should be continued i.e. to avoid prolonged standing and sitting or lying with legs crossed. Encourage the mother to sit with her feet on a stool so that her legs are horizontal or raised slightly higher if oedema is present. Circulatory exercises are helpful at all times but, once the mother is up and about, there are more important exercises to practise if her time is limited.

The Pelvic floor

Pelvic-floor exercises will strengthen the pelvic-floor muscles postnatally with the aim of regaining their full function as soon as possible and helping to prevent any long-term urinary problems or prolapse. However, contraction and relaxation of these muscles will also assist in relieving any discomfort in the perineum which may be present as a result of delivery, and aid healing by promoting local circulation and reducing oedema.

These exercises should be started as soon as possible following delivery to prevent loss of cortical control over the muscles due to perineal pain and apprehension about damaging stitches *(Shepherd, 1980)*. The mother who has had an episiotomy following epidural anaesthesia may feel a sudden intense perineal pain after a painless labour. She may need pain relief to prevent inhibition of the pelvic-floor contraction (see Ch. 7); all mothers must be encouraged to contract their pelvic-floor muscles little and often, slowly and quickly, in the early postpartum period. Postnatally the woman may find the pelvic-floor exercise more difficult because of stretching at delivery and possible discomfort from a bruised or sutured perineum. Plenty of reassurance will be needed as she will probably find she cannot reach the number of contractions she achieved antenatally.

Pelvic-floor exercise

Close the back passage as though preventing a bowel action, close the middle and front passages too as though preventing the flow of urine, then lift up all 3 passages inside. Hold strongly for as long as possible up to 10 seconds, breathing normally throughout. Relax and rest for 3 seconds. Repeat the above **slowly** as many times as possible up to a maximum of 10.

Repeat the exercise lifting and letting go **more quickly** up to 10 times without holding the contraction. The number of repetitions will build up gradually as women will only manage a few initially but must be reassured that this is normal.

By exercising these muscles slowly and quickly, both the slow-twitch and the fast-twitch muscle fibres will be strengthened *(Gilpin et al., 1989)*. The performance of the pelvic-floor exercise can be memory-linked to activities associated with the baby, for example, feeding, bathing, washing. It can be practised whilst sitting on the lavatory **after** each bladder-emptying. This is a relaxed position in which to contract these muscles. A notice can be placed behind the hospital toilet doors as a further reminder. If a painful perineum makes the exercise difficult when sitting, it could be practised in prone, or side-lying positions with a pillow between the legs, or standing with legs slightly apart.

Advice should be given to brace the pelvic floor when coughing, laughing, lifting or squatting down. Mothers should be warned that it could take up to 3 months to regain full pelvic-floor function. However, all women should be encouraged to continue with regular pelvic-floor exercises for the rest of their lives to help prevent future gynaecological problems. They can test the strength of their pelvic-floor muscles 8-12 weeks post delivery by jumping up and down with a full bladder and coughing deeply two or three times while doing so. There should not be any leakage of urine if the muscles have regained their former strength and function. If leakage does occur on testing, the pelvic-floor muscles need further intensive exercising and re-testing 4 weeks later. If there is still leakage, the mother should be referred via her general practitioner to a consultant gynaecologist or an obstetric physiotherapist for specialist treatment. Subsequent pregnancies will only subject the pelvic floor to further strain and should not be undertaken before rehabilitation of the pelvic floor is complete.

For physiotherapeutic treatments to the perineum see Chapter 7.

Abdominal exercises

During pregnancy the abdominal corset has stretched until at term it is approximately twice its original length. All the abdominal muscles will need exercising to regain their former length and strength, and exercises for the straight abdominal muscles - the recti - may be commenced from the first day post-delivery.

Abdominal retraction

Lie on the back with the knees bent and the feet flat on the surface, or sit or stand. Pull in the abdominal muscles and hold for a count of 4, breathing normally. Repeat 5 times. This is a very simple exercise for the abdominals and can be performed frequently in any position.

Pelvic tilting

Lie on the back with the knees bent and the feet flat on the surface. Pull in the abdominal muscles, tighten the muscles of the buttocks and press the small of the back down onto the surface. Hold the position for a count of 4, breathing normally, then relax. Repeat 5 times, building up to 10 or more repetitions over the following 6 weeks. The exercise may also be performed more rhythmically to help to relieve any postural backache which may be present following delivery.

Pelvic tilting should be encouraged in several positions, for instance, sitting and standing may be more convenient than lying when the mother is at home and busy. As with the pelvic-floor exercise, it can be performed in conjunction with many daily activities.

Fig. 8.2 Pelvic tilting exercise

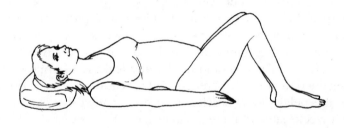

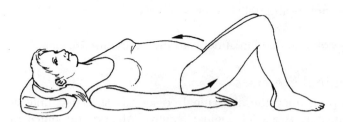

Other abdominal exercises should not be practised before the rectus muscles have been tested to exclude any excessive diastasis. The oblique and transverse muscles are inserted into the linea alba and rectus sheath (see Ch. 1) and diastasis could increase when these muscles are contracted *(Noble, 1988)*. Up to 3cm (2 fingers) width between the rectus muscles is considered acceptable. If the gap is greater than this, rotation and other abdominal exercises should not be performed as the stress on the linea alba may increase the separation.

The midwife is the ideal person to test for diastasis when she is checking the fundus. The mother should lie on her back with one pillow under her head, knees bent up and feet flat on the bed. With the midwife's fingers pressed into the abdomen either just above or below the umbilicus, the mother is asked to lift her head and shoulders off the pillow towards her knees. The rectus muscles will be felt taut either side of the fingers if there is no diastasis. If the rectus muscles cannot be felt until 2 or more fingers are inserted and 'peaking' of the recti is apparent, only pelvic tilting and special diastasis exercises should be commenced (see Ch. 7).

If, on testing, the gap is less than 3cm (2 fingers) or less, it is safe to start the exercises described below for the straight, oblique and transverse abdominal muscles. The exercises will be more effective if performed slowly and the number of repetitions increased according to individual capabilities. It is always better to exercise little and often rather than just once a day. However if the mother is feeling tired or unwell, she should be guided by her body and defer the exercises until she feels better.

Straight curl-ups

Lie on the back with knees bent up, feet flat on the surface, hands on thighs and one pillow under the head. Pull in the abdominal muscles, tilt the pelvis backwards and hold it in this position whilst lifting the head and shoulders forward, sliding the hands towards the knees. Breathe normally, then slowly lower the head and shoulders back onto the pillow before relaxing the pelvic tilt. Repeat 5 times increasing the number of repetitions up to 10 or more over the following six weeks. This exercise must **always** be performed with knees bent and pelvis tilted.

Oblique curl-ups

Lie on the back with the knees bent, the feet flat on the surface, the head on one pillow and arms by the side. Pull in the abdominal muscles, tilt the pelvis backwards and lift the head and shoulders forwards, reaching with the left hand in the direction of the right ankle whilst breathing normally. (The hand may only reach the outside of the opposite knee). Slowly lower back to the pillow and relax the abdominals completely. Change to the left side reaching with the right hand. Repeat 5 times to each side. This can be increased up to 10 repetitions or more to each side by 6 weeks post partum.

Fig. 8.3 Straight curl-up exercise

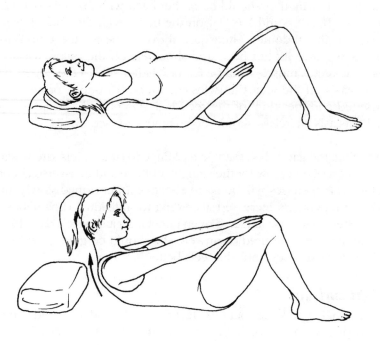

Fig. 8.4 Oblique curl-up exercise

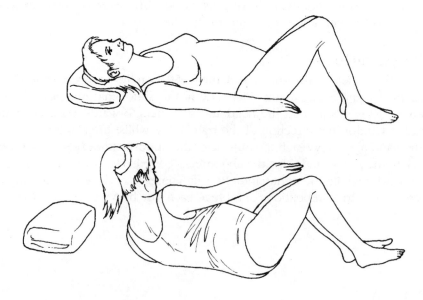

NB. **The abdomen must stay flat throughout these exercises. If there is any 'peaking', the exercise must be stopped.**

Knee rolling

Lie on the back with the knees bent, the feet flat on the surface and arms out to the side to stabilise the trunk. Pull in the abdominal muscles, tilt the pelvis backwards and roll both knees over to the left as far as possible, keeping the shoulders flat on the floor. Return the knees to the centre and relax the abdominals. Pull in the abdominals, pelvic tilt again and repeat the exercise to the right side before returning the knees to the centre and relaxing. This exercise can be repeated up to 5 times to each side progressing up to 10 or more times over the following 6 weeks.

Fig. 8.5 Knee-rolling exercise

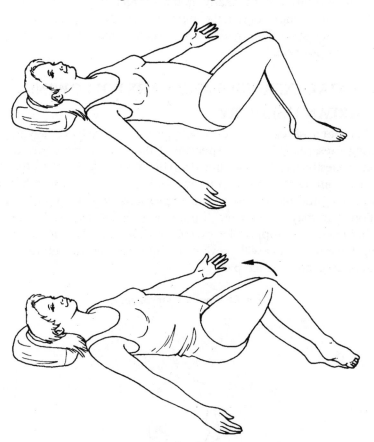

An abdominal exercise known as **hip updrawing** or **hip hitching** is commonly taught postnatally. However, because its action causes the pelvis to tilt laterally, it often causes discomfort over the symphysis and/or sacroiliac joints, particularly if there is undue joint laxity. For this reason, the exercise has been omitted here.

POSTNATAL EXERCISES AND CARE FOLLOWING AN ASSISTED DELIVERY

Mothers who have undergone a forceps delivery or ventouse extraction will have sutures and may have bruising and oedema. These mothers may be reluctant to exercise, but **circulatory** and **pelvic-floor** exercises should be encouraged for their healing effect. **Pelvic tilting** could be started but **other abdominal exercises** may be left until the mother is feeling more comfortable.

Comfortable resting positions are side-lying with a pillow between the legs (see Ch. 4) and prone-lying (many mothers forget they can now lie on their front) with one pillow under the hips and another under the head and shoulders. Breast feeding may be more comfortable in a side-lying rather than a sitting position.

POSTNATAL EXERCISES AND CARE FOLLOWING CAESAREAN DELIVERY

Vigorous **foot and leg** exercises for the circulation are extremely important following caesarean delivery especially if this has been performed under epidural anaesthesia. Two or three deep breaths regularly whilst the mother is relatively immobile will help to improve ventilation. **Deep breathing** followed by "huffing" (short forced expirations) will help to loosen any secretions that may be present. If the mother needs to cough, she should bend her knees and support her wound with her hands or a pillow, whilst leaning forwards. This will prevent undue strain on the sutures, increase her confidence and reduce pain.

Fig. 8.6 Position for coughing

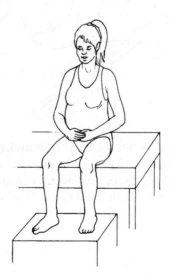

Flatulence is often the cause of great discomfort post-delivery, and may be relieved by gently rolling the knees a few inches to each side (in a "tic - toc" action). **NB. The knees should not be taken far to the sides in case any diastasis of recti is present.**

The mother should be taught how to **move up and down** the bed by bending her knees, pulling in her abdominal muscles and curling forwards whilst pushing on her hands and feet. She will be able to move her body in a forwards or backwards direction. She should not attempt to sit up forwards from a lying position, but instead continue to roll over on to her side as described in Chapter 3. This is also the easiest way of getting out of bed - pulling in the abdominals and pushing up into a sitting position on the edge of the bed.

Pelvic tilting can be commenced whenever the mother feels able. Performed rhythmically, it relieves postural backache resulting from the tilted position on the operating table, and tension in back muscles following an epidural. A check for diastasis of the recti can be done when the mother feels comfortable and other abdominal exercises commenced when the gap is less than 3cm (2 fingers). Progression should be slower than that following a normal delivery.

Pelvic-floor exercises are still important following a caesarean delivery, though if a catheter is in situ, only an occasional contraction should be tried before its removal. It has been demonstrated that it is the pregnancy rather than the delivery that causes the greatest strain on the pelvic-floor muscles *(Francis, 1960)*. The authors have treated several women suffering from urinary problems who have undergone caesarean births only.

Unfortunately, more mothers are having their babies by caesarean delivery and many relatives do not appreciate the fact that these mothers have undergone major surgery and will require more rest and support at home. The midwife will probably find herself answering many questions about when the mother can resume 'normal activities'. Driving is a popular topic and a mother should be advised to check with her insurance company that she is fully covered. When to start also depends on her rate of recovery as she must be able to concentrate fully and perform an emergency stop.

POSTNATAL EXERCISES AND CARE FOLLOWING STILLBIRTH OR NEONATAL DEATH

Women who have had the sad experience of a stillbirth, neonatal death or who have a very ill baby may be cared for in a single room and tend to miss out on postnatal exercises. Special effort needs to be made to offer these women exercises and advice about normal daily activities. They usually prefer to be given this on a one to one basis. A sensitive leaflet should be available which does not refer to the baby eg. feeding, nappy changing.

POSTNATAL CARE OF THE BACK

During the early postnatal period the mother's joints are still unstable because of the hormonal influence on the ligaments and can remain so for up to six months *(Polden and Mantle, 1990)*. The abdominal muscles which help to support the spine and control the pelvic tilt are stretched and weak. So the new mother is at her most vulnerable just when she is faced with so many new activities for the baby which involve bending, stooping or lifting. She is looking forward to being able to resume normal activities and rarely considers possible long-term problems. It is extremely important that the midwife explains the underlying anatomy and physiology to the mother and teaches and/or reinforces awareness of good back care both in hospital and at home. The midwife has the opportunity, when with the mother, to discuss positions for changing and bathing baby which avoid stooping and carrying heavy baths of water. Standing at a surface which is at waist height, or kneeling at a surface which is coffee-table height both obviate the need for stooping whilst carrying out tasks for the baby. The midwife can suggest comfortable and supported positions in which to feed baby so the mother is not bending forward.

Correct posture in all positions will not only alleviate backache, but should also give the mother a sense of good body-image. At first, it will be a matter of re-educating her postural sense in front of a full-length mirror as the brain has got used to the pregnant stance. If she stands sideways to the mirror she will soon see whether her outline is still a semi-pregnant one! However, if the mother checks her posture whenever she stands up, it will soon become a good habit. **Lifting** must be kept to an absolute minimum for the first few weeks if this is at all possible. This is the advice that would be given to a patient with back problems, but it is also relevant in order to prevent problems. However a mother may have to lift if there is no one else to do it for her. In this case she should be encouraged to make the object handled as light as possible and held close to the body. With a little planning, some lifting may be delegated to others. If the mother has no help, the correct lifting procedures as described in Chapter 3 must be followed to avoid back strain at this very vulnerable time. Toddlers should be encouraged to climb onto a chair instead of being lifted, or onto the second or third stair for dressing to avoid the mother stooping.

Fig. 8.7 Positions for feeding, lifting and dressing toddler

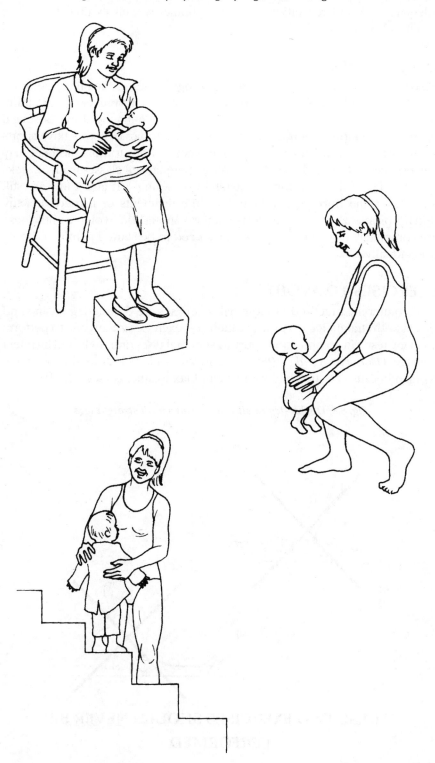

Relatives may need reminding that the newly-delivered mother needs adequate rest and relaxation periods at home as well as time to do her postnatal exercises.

Daily Activities

Heavy housework e.g. vacuuming, moving furniture, cleaning windows should be avoided for several weeks after delivery to prevent back strain. Walking and swimming are good ways of supplementing the above postnatal exercises, but more strenuous keep-fit classes, aerobics or competitive sports should be left for at least ten to twelve weeks. Prior to this, mothers may join especially designed exercise-to-music or aquanatal classes from 6 weeks (see Ch. 11), if they are run by qualified personnel. If any joints are still affected by the hormonal influence on the ligaments or if there are any urinary problems, more strenuous exercise should be avoided until these are completely resolved. New activities need to be started gently and built up gradually.

EXERCISES TO AVOID

Two commonly practised "abdominal" exercises are double-leg raising and sit-ups with straight legs. These are high-risk exercises for anyone to perform and may result in compression injury to vertebral discs or muscle and ligament damage *(Donovan et al., 1988)*. There are added risks to the postnatal woman because of stretched muscles and lax ligaments (see Ch. 7).

Fig. 8.8 Double-leg raising and sit-ups with straight legs

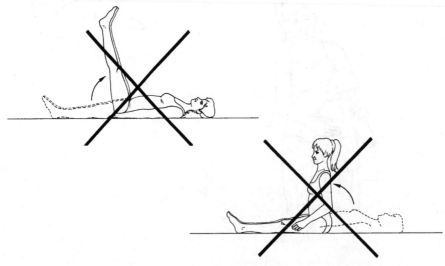

THESE TWO EXERCISES SHOULD <u>NEVER</u> BE PERFORMED

Postnatal Classes

Ideally, mothers should be taught the postnatal exercises in the antenatal period and encouraged to start them as soon as possible in the postnatal period. Unfortunately, many mothers do not attend antenatal classes and will need individually-supervised tuition postnatally. It is very beneficial if group exercises are performed on the postnatal wards, but with many early discharges this is often difficult to arrange. Most midwives will find they are teaching postnatal exercises on a one-to-one basis especially in the home. However, a compromise might be for a postnatal class to be held in the community which mothers could attend when they wished (see Ch. 10). Exercises at these classes could be progressed in strength to include more strenuous activities. The sessions would provide a support network for new mothers and an opportunity for professionals to 'pick up problems.'

References

Donovan G., McNamara J., Gianoli P. *Exercise Danger.* Western Australia: Wellness Australia Pty Ltd. 1988.

Francis W. The onset of stress incontinence. *J. Obst. Gynaecol. Br. Empire.* 1960;67:899

Gilpin S.A., Gosling J.A., Smith A.R.B., Warrell D.W. The pathogenesis of genitourinary prolapse and stress incontinence of urine. A histological and histochemical study. *Brit. J. Obstet. Gynaec.* 1989;96:15

Noble E. *Essential Exercises for the Childbearing Year.* 3rd Edn. Boston:Houghton Mifflin, 1988.

Polden M., Mantle J. *Physiotherapy in Obstetrics and Gynaecology.* Oxford: Butterworth-Heinemann, 1990.

Shepherd A. Re-education of the muscles of the pelvic floor. In: Mandelstam D, Ed. *Incontinence and its Management.* London: Croom Helm, 1980.

Further reading

Fletcher G. *Get Into Shape After Childbirth.* London: Ebury Press, 1991.

Whiteford B. and Polden M. *The Postnatal Exercise Book.* London:Frances Lincoln, 1992.

CHAPTER 9

Teaching Exercises

Physiotherapists specialise in teaching physical skills. It is therefore more difficult for other professionals who are not specifically trained in this field to teach exercises. It is essential that before embarking on this undertaking, the prospective teacher should follow simple guidelines.

She should:
- be proficient at performing the exercises or skills herself
- be completely familiar with the terminology of each exercise or skill
- practise teaching 1 or 2 willing colleagues or family members unfamiliar with the skills
- ask for feedback before attempting to teach a larger group of women/ partners

Several points should be observed when teaching physical skills. The group participants need to know:
- **why** they are learning the particular exercise
- **what** the benefits are
- **how** to perform the exercise correctly
- **when and where** to practise the exercise
- **how many times and how often** to practise
- **additional relevant information and advice**

It must be remembered that in any group 1 or 2 members may have physical problems, for example, lumbar disc lesion, asthma, congenital abnormalities, which could be exacerbated by some exercises or postures. No discomfort should be experienced whilst performing any exercise and the group should be reassured that it is quite permissible to omit a particular exercise or adopt an alternative position if uncomfortable.

Facilities and equipment

Many teachers will find themselves with less than perfect facilities in crowded community clinics. Ideally, the room selected for exercise classes should be private, well ventilated, have plenty of floor and wall space, lighting which can be dimmed and be close to toilets and refreshment facilities.

Chairs of different heights and types would allow posture to be demonstrated in several positions and provide an alternative for the woman who is not comfortable on the floor. A full-length mirror is important to check correct posture in standing.

Mats are desirable but not essential if the room is carpeted. For the exercise and relaxation sessions, each woman should have a right angled wedge which can be either upright against the wall as a backrest for exercises in sitting, or on the floor to allow the woman to be at an angle of 45 degrees when half-lying. In addition 3 pillows would permit her to practise relaxation in different positions. However, pillows can be doubled over, upturned chairs can be used as backrests and women with their own transport are usually willing to bring pillows from home. Failing all of the above suggestions, it may only be possible to demonstrate alternative positions for some activities.

Arranging the group

Ideally, the group should be arranged in a semi-circle or horseshoe so all members can see each other and the educator. Each woman will then feel part of the group and exercises can be checked easily. The teacher should have eye contact with each member of the group whenever possible.

The women will feel less threatened if the teacher is at the same level as themselves i.e. on the floor or on a beanbag rather than standing, though it may be necessary and desirable to move around from time to time. The group should also be encouraged to change position frequently.

The most appropriate **starting position** for each exercise should be selected and the reasons explained to the group. Many exercises can be executed in alternative positions to suit individual needs or to progress the exercise.

The exercises should be introduced one at a time and **described** very clearly using phraseology suitable to the group and/or **demonstrated** before the participants are asked to adopt the starting position. It is not easy to see or hear the instructions when lying down.

Individuals should be aware of the optimum number of **repetitions,** how **frequently** to repeat and how to **progress** each exercise.

The members of the group should be individually **checked** to ensure the exercise is being performed correctly. If the performance is incorrect and allowed to pass unchecked, the woman could cause problems for herself if she continued to practise. Sensitivity must be used to avoid embarrassment to any individual, so a general comment is preferable, though personal correction may still be required.

The group should be encouraged to **practise** regularly at home. Memory-links to suit individuals could be suggested in discussion.

For easy reference, all the exercises described in the antenatal sections are repeated in the postnatal section with the relevant information that should be given to the learner.

The number of repetitions is only approximate for the group as a whole. At all times women should be encouraged to listen to their own bodies and alter the repetitions accordingly.

Sometimes the exercises will be taught just to one woman on her own. Although there will not be the added enjoyment of a group situation, some women prefer this; the explanation being tailored to the woman's individual needs. There will also be women with special needs where exercises may have to be adapted. It may be that all exercise has to be performed in a chair rather than using a mat, or that only part of the routine can be utilised. Often the woman (and partner) will need individual sessions to reinforce the teaching of the exercises but could attend the group as well for support.

The use of music can help to motivate and increase enjoyment and interest in exercise sessions. It can be used with the basic exercises taught both antenatally in preparation for parenthood classes (Ch. 3), and postnatally (Ch. 8). Music with or without beats can be used and classical music is often appropriate. Music should not control and dominate the exercises and it is acceptable to allow pauses during performance when teaching points, instructions and information are given. The teacher will need to emphasise correct execution as the women may be listening to the music and not concentrating on the exercise. During the relaxation period, well-chosen music will help to create a peaceful atmosphere. Music must always be used with care so that a high standard of exercise performance is maintained.

TEACHING THE EXERCISES TO OTHERS

The reader must check that she is fully cognisant of the contents of Chapters 3 and 8 and have confidence in her own performance of each physical skill. She should now be ready to try out the following exercises on 3 or 4 willing colleagues or friends, using the information and instructions on the following pages.

ANTENATAL EXERCISE INSTRUCTIONS AND INFORMATION

FOOT AND LEG EXERCISES

Aim of exercises:

To improve the circulation, particularly the venous return.

Why necessary:

Circulation is slowed because of the
- hormonal influence on vein walls
- increased blood volume
- pressure from enlarged uterus

Sluggish circulation could lead to cramp, swollen ankles and varicose veins.

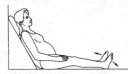

Starting position:

Sitting on the bed, floor or on a chair with the legs stretched out in front and supported.

• *Foot Exercises*

Bend and stretch the ankles briskly.
Repeat at least 10 times.
Circle both feet in as large a circle as possible, keeping the knees still.
Repeat at least 10 times in each direction.

• *Leg tightening*

Pull both feet upwards at the ankle and press the back of the knees down onto the surface. Hold for a count of 4, breathing normally, then relax.
Repeat 5 times.

Frequency:

Whenever possible, particularly early morning, late evening, and when sitting with legs elevated.

Advice:

- sit with legs elevated and supported
- sit instead of standing when possible
- wriggle toes when standing
- don't sit or lie with legs crossed

- wear support tights if necessary
- wear appropriate footwear (see Ch. 3)
- change position frequently
- walking aids circulation

PELVIC-FLOOR EXERCISE

Aim of exercise:

To promote awareness and tone the muscles for pregnancy, labour and the puerperium.

Why necessary:

There is strain on the pelvic floor because of the
- hormonal influence on fascia and muscle
- extra weight of pregnancy
- delivery

Weak muscles could lead to urinary problems, prolapse and sexual problems.

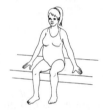

Starting position:

Any comfortable position with the legs slightly apart.

• *Exercise*

Close the back passage as though preventing a bowel action, close the middle and front passages too as though preventing the flow of urine, then lift up all three passages inside. Hold strongly for as long as possible up to 10 seconds, breathing normally throughout.

Relax and rest for 3 seconds.

Repeat the above **slowly** as many times as possible up to a maximum of 10.

Repeat the exercise, lifting up and letting go more **quickly** up to 10 times without holding the contraction.
NB. Make sure you do not tighten the abdominal or buttock muscles.

Frequency:

As many occasions as possible so it becomes a habit. Use a memory-link e.g. after each bladder emptying. Very occasionally test by a "midstream stop".

Advice:

- get into the habit of doing the exercise anywhere, any time
- stop midstream only occasionally
- do not hold breath
- do not tighten abdominals or buttocks
- contract slowly first, then quickly
- refer for professional advice if necessary

PELVIC TILTING

Aim of exercise:

To tone the natural abdominal corset and improve posture and prevent and relieve backache.

Why necessary:

Abdominal muscles are weakened by
- the hormonal effect on muscle and fascia
- the bulk and weight of the uterus
- altered posture

Poor muscle tone could lead to back ache, pelvic arthropathy and dragging lower abdominal pain.

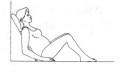

Starting position - lying:

Half-lying at an angle of 45 degrees, supported with a wedge and pillows, with the knees bent up and the feet flat on the surface.

• *Exercise*

Pull in the abdominal muscles, tighten the buttock muscles and press the small of the back down onto the support. Hold for a count of 4, breathing normally, then relax. Repeat 5 times.

Can also be done more rhythmically to ease tension in the back whenever necessary.

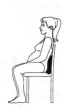

Starting position - supported sitting:

Sitting well back on a dining-type chair with the hands on the knees.

• *Exercise*

Pull in the abdominals, tighten the buttock muscles and press the small of the back into the back of the chair. Hold for a count of 4, breathing normally, then relax. Repeat 5 times.

Starting position - reverse sitting:

Sitting the opposite way round on a chair with the arms round the back of the chair.

• *Exercise*

Pull in the abdominals, tighten the buttock muscles - slightly rounding the lower back - and hold for a count of 4, breathing normally, then relax. Repeat 5 times.

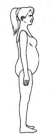

Starting position - standing:

Standing tall with the feet several inches apart and the knees slightly bent.

• *Exercise*

Pull in the abdominal muscles, and tuck in the buttocks. Hold for a count of 4, breathing normally, then relax. Repeat 5 times.

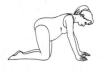

Starting position - prone kneeling:

Kneeling on all fours with the arms and thighs vertical, hands directly under shoulders and knees directly under hips.

• *Exercise*

Pull up the abdominals, tighten the buttock muscles and push the small of the back upwards. Hold for a count of 4, breathing normally, then gently relax the abdominals and allow the spine to flatten - **not hollow**. Repeat 5 times.

Frequency:

Several times a day in the different positions.

Advice:

- the pelvic tilting exercise can also be performed rhythmically (rocking) to relieve backache
- correct standing posture using mirror
- always distribute weight evenly
- refer to an obstetric physiotherapist if there are persistent back problems

POSTNATAL EXERCISE INSTRUCTIONS AND INFORMATION

FOOT AND LEG EXERCISES
Aim of exercises:
To improve the circulation, particularly venous return.

Why necessary:
Circulation is slowed, especially after epidural or general anaesthesia, because of the
  - hormonal influences of pregnancy
  - loss of fluid at delivery
  - increased waste products
  - decreased intra-abdominal pressure
  - relative immobility

Slowed circulation could lead to deep venous thrombosis, swollen ankles, pulmonary embolus or discomfort in legs.

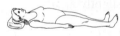

Starting position:
Lying or sitting on the bed, floor or chair with the legs stretched out in front and supported.

• *Foot Exercises*
Bend and stretch the ankles briskly.
Repeat at least 10 times.
Circle both feet in as large a circle as possible, keeping the knees still.
Repeat at least 10 times in each direction.

• *Leg tightening*
Pull both feet upwards at the ankle and press the back of the knees down onto the surface. Hold for a count of 4, breathing normally, then relax.
Repeat 5 times.

Frequency:
Whenever possible, particularly early morning, late evening, and when sitting with the legs elevated.

Advice:
- sit with legs elevated and supported
- sit instead of standing when possible
- wriggle toes when standing
- do not sit or lie with legs crossed
- change position frequently
- walking aids circulation

PELVIC-FLOOR EXERCISE

Aim of exercise:
To re-educate and strengthen the muscles and promote healing.

Why necessary:
The weakening of the pelvic floor by the strain of pregnancy or trauma of delivery can lead to urinary and sexual problems and prolapse.

Starting position:
Any comfortable position with legs slightly apart.

• *Exercise*
Close the back passage as though preventing a bowel action, close the middle and front passages too as though preventing the flow of urine, then lift up all three passages inside. Hold strongly for as long as possible up to a maximum of 10 seconds, breathing normally throughout. Relax and rest for 3 seconds.

Repeat the above **slowly** as many times as you can up to a maximum of 10.

Repeat the exercise, lifting up and letting go **more quickly** up to 10 times without holding the contraction.

NB. **Make sure you do not tighten the abdominal or buttock muscles.**

Frequency:
As many occasions as possible so it becomes a habit. Use a memory-link e.g. after each bladder emptying. Very occasionally test by "a midstream stop".

Link the pelvic-floor exercise to activities with the baby.

Advice:

- get into the habit - anywhere, any time
- stop midstream only occasionally
- do not hold breath
- do not tighten abdominals or buttocks
- contract slowly first, then quickly
- test strength at 8-12 weeks (see Ch. 8)
- refer for professional advice if necessary

ABDOMINAL EXERCISES

Aim of exercises:

To strengthen the abdominal muscles and regain full function of the natural muscular corset.

Why necessary:

Abdominal muscles are weakened by the hormonal influences of pregnancy and stretching of the muscles; this could lead to long term back problems, lack of support, poor figure and loss of self-esteem.

PELVIC TILTING

Starting position - lying:

Lying with the knees bent up and the feet flat on the bed or the floor.

•Exercise

Pull in the abdominal muscles, tighten the buttock muscles and press the small of the back down onto the support. Hold for a count of 4, breathing normally, then relax. Repeat 5 times. This can also be done more rhythmically to ease tension in the back whenever necessary.

Starting position - supported sitting:

Sitting well back on a dining-type chair with the hands resting on the knees.

•Exercise

Pull in the abdominals, tighten the buttock muscles and press the small of the back into the back of the chair. Hold for a count of 4, breathing normally, then relax. Repeat 5 times.

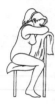

Starting position - reverse sitting:

Sitting the opposite way round on a chair with the arms round the back of the chair

• *Exercise*

Pull in the abdominals, tighten the buttock muscles - slightly rounding the lower back - and hold for a count of 4, breathing normally, then relax. Repeat 5 times.

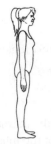

Starting position - standing:

Standing tall with feet several inches apart and knees slightly bent.

• *Exercise*

Pull in the abdominal muscles and tuck in the buttocks. Hold for a count of 4, breathing normally, then relax. Repeat 5 times.

Frequency:

Several times a day in the different positions.

Advice:

- the pelvic tilting exercise can also be performed rhythmically (rocking) to relieve backache
- correct standing posture using mirror
- always distribute weight evenly
- refer to an obstetric physiotherapist if there are persistent back problems

STRAIGHT CURL-UPS

NB. This exercise should only be performed when no significant diastasis is detected (see Ch. 7)

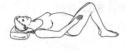

Starting position:

Lying with the knees bent, the feet flat on the surface and the hands resting on the thighs.

• *Exercise*

Pull in the abdominals, tilt the pelvis backwards, lift the head and shoulders, curling forwards to reach towards the knees with the hands. Lower back slowly, breathing normally. Repeat 5 times slowly.

OBLIQUE CURL-UPS

NB. This exercise should only be performed when no significant diastasis is detected (see Ch. 7).

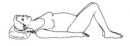

Starting position:

Lying with the knees bent, the feet flat on the surface and the arms by the side.

• *Exercise*

Pull in the abdominals, tilt the pelvis back, lift the head and shoulders, curling forwards to reach with one hand in the direction of the opposite ankle. (Hand may only reach outside of opposite knee). Lower back slowly. Breathe normally throughout. Repeat this exercise 5 times to each side.

NB. The abdomen must stay flat throughout these exercises, if there is any 'peaking', the exercise must be stopped.

KNEE ROLLING

NB. This exercise should only be performed when no significant diastasis is detected (see Ch. 7)

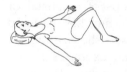

Starting position:

Lying with the knees bent, the feet flat on the surface and the arms out to the side.

• *Exercise*

Pull in the abdominals, tilt the pelvis backwards and keeping both knees together, roll them over to the right as far as is comfortable. Bring the knees back to the centre, then relax the abdominals. Breathe normally throughout. Repeat 5 times to each side.

Frequency:

Morning and evening.

Advice:

- all the abdominal exercises should be performed slowly
- check starting position is correct, knees should

always be bent when performing straight and oblique curl-ups or pelvic tilting in lying
- always lift the head and shoulders together
- the abdomen must always remain flat whilst performing abdominal exercises
- don't hold breath whilst exercising
- stop if it hurts - Pain does not mean gain!

These abdominal exercises may be progressed by gradually increasing the number of repetitions or frequency of performance. Straight or oblique curl ups can be made more difficult by removing the pillow from under the head before performing the exercise.

DOUBLE-LEG RAISING AND SIT-UPS WITH STRAIGHT LEGS SHOULD <u>NEVER</u> BE PERFORMED.

Evaluation of teaching

It is now time for the educator to evaluate her performance as a teacher of these basic physical skills. Did the feedback indicate that all the relevant teaching points had been included? Does the reader feel more confident? Is further practice needed before introducing these skills to groups of antenatal or postnatal women? When the educator has mastered the teaching of the basic exercises, she may like to include the following additional exercises in her preparation for parenthood programme. These are chosen for the pregnant woman and are not appropriate postnatally.

ADDITIONAL ANTENATAL EXERCISES

SHOULDER, ARM AND CHEST EXERCISES

Aim of exercises:

To tone the shoulder and pectoral muscles and relieve upper backache and pressure in the shoulder region and upper ribs.

Why necessary:

Kyphosis often occurs in pregnancy and may cause aching on shoulders and upper back.

Rib flare causes pressure under the ribs.

Oedema causes pressure which could lead to tingling in fingers and in the shoulder region.

Breasts increase in size and weight and require increased support.

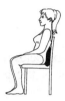

Starting position:

Sitting on chair with back well supported or tailor-sitting

• *Exercises*

1. Raise and lower both shoulders together slowly. Repeat 5-10 times.

2. Rest fingers on shoulders. Slowly and rhythmically bring both elbows forwards, upwards, backwards and then down, making large backward circles with the elbows. Repeat 5-10 times.

3. Slowly stretch the right arm above the head and lower. Do the same with the left arm. Repeat 5-10 times. An added lift is gained if the trunk is bent very slightly to the opposite side while stretching.

4. Lift elbows to shoulder height. Make a loose fist with one hand and clasp the other round it. Slowly press hands together and release. Repeat this exercise 5-10 times. Change hands and repeat.

Frequency

Once/twice per day.

Advice:

-   breathe easily during exercises.
-   do not arch the lower back during these exercises.
-   be aware of posture of upper back and so avoid slumping (slouching) forwards.

STRETCHING EXERCISES

WARNING: Stretching exercises should always be preceded by warm-up exercises, and pregnant women must NEVER overstretch.

Aim of exercises:

To prepare women physically and psychologically for taking up and holding wide advantageous positions for labour and delivery.

Why necessary:

There is shortness and tightness of the muscles of the calves and inner thighs and ligaments of the groin, hips and lower limbs.

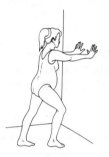

Starting position:

Standing at arm's length from a wall (**not a door**) with palms pressed against it, one foot behind the other.

•*Exercise*

Lean gently into the wall, bending the front leg and both elbows slightly. A stretch in the calf muscle will be felt in the back leg. Hold the stretch for half to one minute.

Change legs and repeat. If this feels very easy, move the back leg further apart away from the other leg.

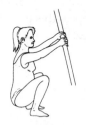

Starting position:

Squatting, holding on to a firm support or partner.

•*Exercise*

Practise holding this position for half a minute and gradually increase to one minute.

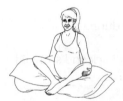

Starting Position:

Sitting on the floor with the back supported and the soles of the feet together, knees resting on a pillow.

•*Exercise*

Keep the feet as close to the pelvis as possible and hold the position for as long as you are comfortable.

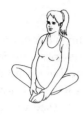

Starting position:

Sitting on floor with the back supported and the soles of the feet together, hands holding ankles and feet pulled in towards the perineum.

•*Exercise*

Allow the weight of the legs to take the knees down towards the floor for half a minute and gradually increase to one minute.

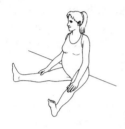

Starting position:

Sitting with the back supported and the legs out in front and wide apart, keeping the knees straight.

•*Exercise*

Pull the feet up towards the body at the ankle, without bending the knees. Hold the stretch for half a minute increasing to one minute.

Frequency:

Once/twice per day

Advice:

- remember to warm up the body
- always repeat stretches slowly
- at first a point will be reached where the stretch is felt; breathe easily until the sensation ceases staying with the stretch
- the range of movement will gradually be increased and the body will feel more flexible and relaxed
- never force movements
- the squatting position may only be able to be held with heels off the ground at first
- follow stretching with a warm bath or shower

WARNING

These stretching exercises should not be practised if any pain is experienced in the symphysis pubis area as this might indicate separation at the joint (see Ch. 2). Caution should also be taken if there is any backache and exercises stopped if any pain is felt. Stretches should **NEVER** be developed (forced) during pregnancy because of the laxity of ligaments (see Ch. 2).

Further advice

It is always better to advise women to exercise for a short period regularly, rather than for longer less frequent sessions. They should not exercise when feeling tired or unwell, and should build up gradually after a break from exercising. Individuals will progress at different rates, depending on pre-pregnancy fitness, age, delivery and parity and should exercise to suit their personal needs and comfort.

CHAPTER 10

Programme Planning for Physical Skills

THE ANTENATAL TEAM

The composition of the antenatal education team will vary in different centres. Ideally it consists of a midwife, a health visitor and an obstetric physiotherapist. An obstetrician, anaesthetist, NCT teacher, dietitian and social worker may be involved for occasional talks during the series. Outside speakers may also be invited to special meetings to discuss such subjects as car safety seats, toys and feeding. Parents who have recently given birth may be invited to share their experiences.

An obstetric physiotherapist is the professional with the knowledge and expertise to teach the physical skills input to antenatal groups (see Tripartite Agreement page 6). Physiotherapists specialising in obstetrics are in short supply and, if one is not available, the midwife or health visitor may be required to teach exercises, relaxation and coping strategies for labour.

This chapter only intends to make suggestions as to types of classes where physical skills are appropriate, and outlines the content of these skills for each type of class. It will not discuss parentcraft topics.

There can be no fixed standard scheme of antenatal education. Choice of type of classes, content, length, time, numbers, leaders and venue will all depend on local, economic, and social factors and will vary considerably from place to place. Discussion with the women and their partners should always take place at the start of any programme to ascertain what the group would like included in the course. They always request breathing and relaxation and often ask how to relieve discomforts in pregnancy.

Health and safety precautions should always be considered when choosing both venue and optimum numbers for an antenatal group which will be performing exercises and relaxation. Classes which are too large do not allow the teacher to supervise individually or observe women who may be looking uncomfortable, nor do they allow space for exercises or relaxation to be practised effectively. It is suggested that 8 to 12 in a group works well and allows for the fostering of close personal relationships which can add to the clients' satisfaction *(Wilson, 1990)*. It would be ideal for 2 members of the antenatal team to lead a 2-hour session together, but this may not be economically possible. If just one professional is with the group at any one time, another person should be nearby in case of emergency.

Security is important in community clinics, particularly at night, and this aspect may influence the choice of venue for an evening course.

PHYSICAL SKILLS CONTENT OF ANTENATAL CLASSES

Early Pregnancy

The hormonal effects on the musculoskeletal system occur very early in pregnancy (see Ch. 2), so it makes sense to encourage couples to attend early pregnancy classes, e.g. at about 12 weeks. Combes and Schonveld(1992) suggest that it is most appropriate to cover health and lifestyle issues in the first three months of pregnancy when they are most significant for the health of the mother and baby. However, in practice the woman is often extremely tired at this stage and may still be feeling nauseous. Her partner may only just be coming to terms with the fact that he is to become a father. These factors often mean that attendances at this time are low. Inviting couples to evening sessions a little later, e.g. at about 16 weeks, usually results in a better attendance. Unfortunately, resources often limit this early session to a 'one-off', whereas two or three sessions would allow time for information to be assimilated at a reasonable pace and give the parents-to-be the opportunity to ask questions.

If there is only one evening allocated, then the desirable physical skills input would be a discussion and demonstration/practice of comfortable postures in all positions, both resting and working, correct handling and lifting techniques, pelvic tilting, pelvic-floor and circulatory exercises. If the numbers are large, the exercises may have to be performed on chairs, but it should always be possible to demonstrate other positions. Advice on sufficient rest and delegation of chores should be included and if a second evening is available, relaxation would be the obvious addition to the above. It is very much easier to learn pelvic tilting and pelvic-floor exercises at this stage of pregnancy than later. Prevention of backache and postural problems is very much better than cure *(Mantle et al., 1981)*.

Sometimes these early-pregnancy evenings are more popular in local clinics so that couples do not have to travel to a central hospital.

Women only

These classes usually take place during the daytime from about 30-32 weeks of pregnancy when many women have finished work. A 2-hour session allows time for practising physical skills, comfort breaks and refreshments, parentcraft discussions, demonstrations and/or visits. Classes often lead to friendships and local support groups which last throughout early parenthood.

A preparation for parenthood course commonly consists of 5-8 two-hour sessions. At the first session, it must be established whether anyone has any physical problems, for example, long-term back pain, asthma, which could possibly be exacerbated by different positions. These women must always understand that they are free to omit any position or activity with which they are not comfortable, or to try an alternative.

During the first session, discussing the musculoskeletal and circulatory changes occurring during pregnancy will lead on to the need for good backcare and exercises to prevent long term problems in the future. Foot and leg exercises, pelvic tilting and discussion and experimentation with comfortable and practical postures for daily activities could all be included in this session. The group will volunteer positions and situations of stress when this topic is discussed and a chosen technique of relaxation can be introduced. Many physiotherapists and midwives prefer the physiological relaxation described in Chapter 4, but if a woman has her own method of relaxation, she could continue using it. Breathing awareness is a logical accompaniment to relaxation. The group can discuss opportunities for the practice of relaxation. It is not good use of the professional's time to let the group spend too long relaxing during the class unless it is a convenient time for her to go and make the tea! However the women should need no exhorting to practice the relaxation technique at home. Relaxation in different positions, correct lifting and posture should be practised in every session.

It may be better to introduce the pelvic floor in the second session rather than in the first, as sufficient time is needed to emphasise its importance and to practise the exercise. Members of the group can suggest memory-links and suitable times and situations to practise at home and at work.

The next two or three sessions will cover labour and could include positions of ease for first stage, relaxation, breathing awareness and adaptations when necessary (see Ch. 5), massage, pain relief (including a demonstration and practice with TENS), practical positions for second stage, alternative positions for delivery and the role of the partner. Ideally, these sessions will link in with topics previously covered in the parentcraft programme. The women appreciate at least one evening session during the course to which they can bring their partners to rehearse labour, visit the delivery suite, neonatal unit and postnatal wards, and maybe watch a relevant video.

The postnatal scene could be considered in the last session. Postnatal exercises, the need for adequate rest and relaxation, posture, lifting, resuming normal and sporting activities are all topics which could be discussed at this time. The group should be taught how to check for diastasis recti postnatally. They should be told that, if they are worried, they should seek the advice of their obstetric physiotherapist or midwife. Stronger and rotational abdominal exercises can be demonstrated to the group at this last session and an illustrated postnatal programme given out as a reminder.

Some women will prefer not to attend classes for social or economic reasons, but antenatal preparation can be given on a one-to-one basis in clinic or at home by the midwife. Any woman with **special needs** because of a permanent or temporary disability should be referred to an obstetric physiotherapist if at all possible. She will require individual assessment and, depending on her needs, adaptations of supports, starting positions or exercises may allow the woman to join in the regular antenatal sessions. It may be more appropriate, however, for advice and instruction to be continued on an individual basis in the local clinic or the woman's own home.

Couples

In many areas the demand for couples classes has increased so dramatically over the last few years that mornings/afternoons for women only are relatively few. Even though many men are allowed time off by liberated employers for antenatal classes, the preference for evening or weekend sessions far outweighs that for daytime classes. It was found that half the men attending just one evening session with their partners did not find it very enjoyable *(Hassey, 1990)*. They wanted to be able to attend all the classes with their partners as the one class did not give sufficient time.

When a whole series of couples classes is offered, the men enjoy joining in the exercises and relaxation and should be encouraged to do so, rather than watching. If space is at a premium, they may have to perform the exercises in alternative positions. The couples can practise relaxation and coping strategies for labour in pairs and, where wedges and pillows are in short supply, the men can act as backrests and supports for different positions. Practical massage sessions are both fun and beneficial. The men will learn a skill with which they can help their partners both during pregnancy and labour. The role of the supporter in labour can be discussed as can worries expressed by both partners. Often, the couples gain from separating for part of the evening to allow different topics to be discussed by the men or women separately.

Caesarean delivery

In areas with a high rate of caesarean deliveries it is worth considering devoting classes solely to mothers who will be having an elective caesarean birth. In a survey held to evaluate consumer satisfaction of antenatal classes, only 18% of those who had undergone a caesarean delivery were satisfied with the antenatal preparation they received *(Hassey, 1990)*.

These women and their partners will not be as interested in adaptations of breathing for late first and second stage, but will want to know the pros and cons of epidural versus general anaesthesia and more about the actual procedure. The mothers will need to learn how to move up and down and in and out of bed after delivery (see Ch. 8), without increasing pain. Circulatory exercises immediately following pelvic surgery are extremely important, especially after epidural or spinal anaesthesia, as there will be increased fluid and the leg muscles may feel lethargic. Positions for coughing, feeding and other activities with the baby can be demonstrated and practised.

Partners and relatives may need reminding that a caesarean delivery is not 'the easy way out'. Instead, they have to recognise that the mother has undergone major surgery in addition to giving birth and that she will take longer to recuperate than a woman who has had a vaginal delivery. Practical advice about resuming activities such as driving, housework may be discussed now, so the couple can plan for extra help if this is possible (see Ch. 8).

Transcutaneous electrical nerve stimulation

If the demand is sufficient, it is appropriate to arrange a special time for couples who are interested in using transcutaneous electrical nerve stimulation in labour (see Ch. 6). Women should experience its effects before deciding that they would like to use it in labour as occasionally a woman finds she does not find the sensation comfortable. A video illustrating the way the obstetric TENS works will save technical explanations. Different models can be demonstrated and the advantages discussed before the couple decide whether or not to hire one (see Ch. 6). Some delivery suites have sufficient TENS units to be able to lend one to a couple before the birth, or have a rental scheme in operation. However, many couples choose to hire their own. Partners should be taught where and how to site the electrodes and supervised doing this if possible.

Ethnic minorities

In some areas with high ethnic minority populations, it may be desirable to hold special classes for these women. An interpreter or link worker can be employed, but it may not be possible to translate directly as certain English phrases and explanations are unacceptable to other cultures. Alternative descriptions need to be discussed with a professional who could help with this. The extended family is much more widespread in some of these communities and it may be necessary to gain the confidence and encouragement of the female head of the family before inviting the women to attend classes. Handouts cannot be directly translated into other languages because of the different acceptable terminology and professional advice must be sought before preparing leaflets for ethnic minorities. Another problem is the number of dialects which exist in any one language, making it impossible to include all of them. Many women are not encouraged to participate fully in everyday activities, and some may not be able to read. If an interpreter is used, it should always be a female, as some of these women are not willing to discuss anything related to sex - even pelvic-floor exercises -with a male. Occasionally, it may be appropriate for a midwife or health visitor to hold a group session in the home of one of the group members.

Teenagers' clubs

Teenagers' clubs or groups fulfil a very real need as long as they provide a relaxed atmosphere where the girls feel they can "do their own thing" with no pressure to conform. Organisers should not be discouraged if the girls do not attend regularly, but just drop in when they feel like it. A companion of either sex should be invited to accompany the teenager. A loosely structured programme is all that is possible *(Will, 1990, Evans and Parker, 1985)*, and it has been found that the teenagers are very reluctant to join in any exercises at all, though relaxation has slightly more appeal *(Todd et al., 1988)*. Hopefully, demonstrations of positions and coping strategies for labour will be recalled when needed, even though they have not been practised.

Refreshers

Refresher classes for multiparous women may include physical skills only, if the mothers feel they are happy about baby care. Sessions can be held for one or two hours as a one-off or as a series over 3-4 weeks, and can cover anything the mothers request. Usually they ask for relaxation and breathing. Sometimes the mothers have delivered at home or in other units and welcome the opportunity for a visit to the delivery suite where are booked to have their baby. Mothers who have longer gaps between pregnancies and no ties with toddlers often prefer to attend a full course with first-time mothers. They may have either forgotten parentcraft techniques, or need updating as newer ideas have emerged since their last delivery. These women can be a valuable addition to the classes especially in discussion on postnatal activities.

Ward classes

When women have been admitted to the antenatal ward during their pregnancy, they have plenty of time to discuss parentcraft topics and learn such physical skills as are safe to practise even if bed rest has been advised. Relaxation will always be beneficial and a good time to hold a group session would be just before the afternoon rest period. If the woman is confined to bed, foot and leg exercises are essential to prevent circulatory stasis, particularly if there is oedema present due to hypertension. If the woman is able to join the regular antenatal class, she will enjoy the change from the ward atmosphere as well as learning new skills.

POSTNATAL CLASSES

In these days of early discharges and demand-feeding, it is very difficult to arrange group postnatal classes in hospital. This is a pity as they can be fun and motivate the mothers to practise their exercises. Ideally, all women should receive individual postnatal exercise instruction and advice before leaving hospital. With current restraints, however, this is not always possible and the onus is falling increasingly on the midwife to provide this service when the woman has been transferred home.

Community postnatal classes

Some authorities run postnatal exercise classes in the community along similar lines to antenatal classes. Mothers can attend at weekly intervals for as long as they wish and babies are invited too! Exercises are progressed, preparing mothers to return to more strenuous sporting activities. Examples of stronger postnatal exercises can be found in the further reading at the end of Chapter 8.

Postnatal reunion

The provision of a monthly reunion class allows a group of mothers and their babies to meet up with each other and the antenatal teachers approximately 6 weeks after the last mother in the group was due to deliver. It is a forum for general exchange of notes and ideas, where any physical problems or anxieties can be brought up. By this time any backache or urinary problems should have subsided but, if not, the mother can be referred on to an obstetric physiotherapist. It might also be at this time that the woman is aware of dyspareunia, which can also be treated by an obstetric physiotherapist (see Ch. 7). The reunion may be purely a social and problem-airing session or could include a revision of postnatal exercises, baby-massage and suggestions for future activities. The postnatal reunion is also an ideal opportunity for the evaluation of the preparation for parenthood sessions attended by the group. Combes and Schonveld(1992) state that more attention could be given to the provision of support groups during the first six weeks, and after the first four or five months postnatally.

References

Combes G., Schonveld A. Life will never be the same again. London: Health Education Authority. 1992

Evans G., Parker P. Preparing teenagers for parenthood. *Midwives Chronicle.* 1985;vol.98,1172:239

Hassey L. An evaluation of antenatal classes. *Journal of The Association of Chartered Physiotherapists in Obstetrics and Gynaecology.* 1990;67:17.

Mantle M.J., Holmes J., Currey H.L.F. Backache in pregnancy 11: Prophylactic Influence of Back Care Classes. *Rheum. Rehab.* 1981;20:227

Todd J.E., Lapthorn J., McIntosh J. Teenage Club at the Royal Berkshire. *Midwives Chronicle.* 1988;vol.101,1207:238

Will A. A physiotherapist's view of teenage antenatal classes. *Journal of The Association of Chartered Physiotherapists in Obstetrics and Gynaecology.* 1990;67:15

Wilson P. *Antenatal Teaching.* London: Faber & Faber, 1990.

Further reading

Campion M.J. *The Baby Challenge: a handbook on pregnancy for women with a physical disability.* London: Routledge, 1990.

Rooke J. Cultural differences in pregnancy. *Journal of The Association of Chartered Physiotherapists in Obstetrics and Gynaecology.* 1991;69:7

Wilson P. *Antenatal Teaching.* London: Faber & Faber, 1990.

CHAPTER 11

Alternative Approaches to Fitness

The exercise content of preparation for parenthood programmes (see Ch. 3) is generally limited and many women are now requesting guidance on further exercise. It has been noted that nearly 45% of women of childbearing age exercise *(Sady and Carpenter, 1989)*. When pregnant, many of these wish to continue. Women who do not normally exercise often become more health-conscious in pregnancy. Women ask if it is safe to exercise, they want to know what sport can be continued and hope to benefit using safe but effective exercises during pregnancy.

Changes take place in the body during pregnancy and can affect exercise performance. The heart rate and stroke volume are already increased *(Bush, 1992)*, and will increase further during exercise. The respiratory centre is more sensitive to carbon dioxide so the woman becomes increasingly breathless. There is an increase in weight and the effect of relaxin has made ligaments more pliable, the joints becoming less stable. As the uterus becomes larger, there is an increase in lumbar lordosis and the pelvis is tilted forwards. The woman is less nimble and she can lose balance more easily (see Ch. 2). These factors can lead to the woman being more prone to musculoskeletal injury.

The benefits of exercise are well-known. There is a build-up of endurance so the pregnant woman is more comfortable and capable and her muscle tone and cardiovascular and respiratory function are improved. There is an increase in body-awareness and posture is improved. As the woman adapts to her increase in weight and changing balance, she protects herself against muscle injury, joint strain and backache *(Jacobson et al., 1991)*. Women who take moderate regular exercise during pregnancy are more likely to have an improved course of pregnancy and labour when compared with those leading a sedentary lifestyle *(Huch and Erkkola, 1990, Clapp, 1990)*.

Just as in non-pregnant exercisers, there are also physical and psychological effects for the pregnant woman. It has been shown statistically that there was higher esteem and lower physical discomfort amongst pregnant women who exercised regularly than in those who did not exercise *(Wallace et al., 1986)*. The woman will have an improved body-image and appearance and she will feel fitter. She will sleep better and so have an increased sense of well-being and be less fatigued.

Many women hope that their fitness will help them during labour and delivery and expedite postnatal recovery. It has been found that women who continued to exercise during pregnancy had a lower incidence of abdominal and vaginal operative delivery, and active labour was shorter in those who were delivered vaginally *(Clapp, 1990)*. It is generally accepted that physically-fit women recover more quickly after the birth *(Polden and Mantle, 1990)*.

What advice should be given to these women and what can be offered to them? Provided that there is no obstetric problem or pre-existing disease, moderate aerobic exercise is safe *(Wallace et al., 1986)*. However, women should not take up anything new which is strenuous during pregnancy. It has been stated that a healthy pregnant woman can afford a constant amount of physical activity during the first and second trimesters, but a modest reduction of the training programme would be wise during the last trimester *(Revelli et al., 1992)*. The types of exercise which provide the best cardiovascular and psychological benefits during pregnancy include walking, cycling and swimming.

A moderate aerobic programme would be 30 minutes, 3 days per week with the heart rate not exceeding 150 beats per minute *(Sady et al., 1989)*. However, more recently 60 minutes of physical activity 3 days per week with an intensity which keeps the heart rate under 120 to 130 beats per minute has been recommended *(Revelli et al., 1992)*. Some exercise, for example, high-impact aerobics, and any contact sport or physical activities involving sudden starts and changes of direction, e.g. tennis or basketball, are contraindicated during pregnancy. Any sport where there is risk of an abdominal blow or breast trauma should be avoided and downhill skiing is a poor choice for the woman in late pregnancy *(Revelli et al., 1992)*. It is suggested that water-skiing and scuba-diving could be potentially hazardous and that learning a new sport during pregnancy is inadvisable *(Sady et al., 1989)*; dehydration and fatigue should be avoided. Women who normally horse-ride need to be warned about the risk of a fall and possible stress to the sacroiliac joint and spine. A gentle hack is safer and more sensible than more strenuous activities. With all types of sport and exercise, competition is generally inadvisable during pregnancy because of the anxiety and maximal efforts imposed *(Revelli et al., 1992)*.

It is advised that women should avoid hyperthermia throughout pregnancy since it could be injurious to the fetus *(Huch and Erkkola, 1990)*. During the first trimester, raised maternal core temperatures may bring about teratogenic effects *(Polden and Mantle, 1990)*. It is also suggested by Polden and Mantle that intensive exercise during pregnancy might result in intrauterine growth retardation, preterm labour and, due to redistribution of blood flow, fetal distress.

Because of the demand for exercise in pregnancy and the postnatal period, specially designed exercise-to-music and aquanatal classes are now available. Care must be taken to direct pregnant women only to those aquanatal and antenatal/postnatal exercise-to-music classes which are taken by **qualified** teachers. They can provide expert advice and specially selected exercises for pregnancy and the postnatal period. Classes are suitable for women, whether they are used to exercise or not, because they are low-impact and not over-exerting and are tailored to the individual's needs. They will increase body-awareness and maintain mobility and tone but are not aimed at increasing fitness levels; pregnancy is not the time to try to do this. These sessions offer group support and extra care is taken of the woman. Antenatally they would supplement rather than replace preparation for parenthood classes.

Safety is of paramount importance and it is vital to screen each woman before she starts exercising *(Ashton, 1992)*. Medical clearance should be obtained. The contraindications to exercise in pregnancy include such disorders of pregnancy as threatened miscarriage, preterm labour, uterine haemorrhage, pre-eclampsia or intra-uterine growth retardation *(Huch and Erkkola, 1990)*. Exercise is also contraindicated for women suffering from significant valvular or ischaemic heart disease, type 1 diabetes mellitus, peripheral vascular disease, uncontrolled hypertension and thyroid disease *(Wolfe et al., 1989)*. Physical work must also be especially limited in multiple pregnancy, rupture of membranes, placenta praevia and in women with respiratory illness *(Revelli et al., 1992)*. Screening should also include checking for musculoskeletal problems, for example, diastasis symphysis pubis, sacroiliac strain, backache and continence problems.

Every exercising woman should stop exercising immediately if one of the following symptoms appears: vaginal bleeding, abdominal pain, severe tachycardia, chest pain, severe breathlessness, headache, loss of muscle control, dizziness, nausea. The woman must consult her obstetrician if any of these occur *(Revelli et al., 1992)*.

EXERCISE-TO-MUSIC

Antenatal
An antenatal exercise-to-music programme begins with a warm-up session and short stretch. This can be followed by a gentle/moderate aerobic section

designed to suit the woman's needs, muscle strengthening, stretching, cool-down and relaxation. Some floor work would be included. It is suggested that the aerobic section lasts for no more than 15 minutes *(Artal and Wiswell, 1986)*. There should be no bouncy, jerky movements, no full extension or flexion of joints, and no quick changes of direction because of the compromised balance mentioned earlier. Breath-holding must be discouraged to prevent rise in intra-abdominal pressure, and muscle work needs to be varied.

The women will need to alter their level of exercise according to their stage of pregnancy (see above). Any exercise (or relaxation) normally performed lying flat on the back should be executed in a modified position after the fourth month of pregnancy because of the risk of developing the supine hypotensive syndrome (see Ch. 2).

The exercises include those which are especially relevant for the pregnant woman; pelvic tilting, pelvic-floor and stretching. The aim and advantage of each should be explained with emphasis on good technique, poise and posture in all movements. Concepts of good back care are also introduced. Particular care will be taken by a qualified instructor to avoid the inclusion of exercises which could be harmful for the pregnant woman, for instance, wide deep squats, lumbar extension. An active cool-down is especially important for the pregnant woman because venous pooling might occur with abrupt cessation of activity and venous return may already be hampered by the growing uterus *(Sady and Carpenter, 1989)*. A session would last for approximately 45 minutes and finish with relaxation.

It is not wise to exercise directly after a meal. It could be suggested that the women eat a light carbohydrate-rich snack about one hour before the start of the session.

Postnatal

Postnatally, the mothers usually return to exercise-to-music sessions from about 6 weeks following delivery. It is advised that, on average, mothers who have not exercised before pregnancy join the postnatal group at 9 weeks post delivery *(Ashton, 1992)*. Consideration must be given to the physical changes which took place during pregnancy, remembering that joints are still vulnerable and the pelvic floor and abdominal muscles may still be weak (see Ch. 7).

Screening is again essential and should include checking if there are any pelvic-floor (continence), back or symphysis pubis problems and women referred to an obstetric physiotherapist if necessary. The abdomen should be palpated for possible diastasis of the rectus abdominis muscles before proceeding to abdominal work (see Chs. 7 and 8).

The programme for the postnatal session can be similar to that run antenatally. Exercise is adapted to suit the mother's individual needs and ability. The class can last up to an hour and may include a little more aerobic work and more strengthening exercises especially of the pelvic-floor and abdominal muscles. Again there is emphasis on good posture and back care. Finishing with relaxation is particularly relevant for this group.

Facilities and equipment

A large well-ventilated room is required with a non-slip floor surface e.g. wood or carpet. Cloakrooms with toilets should be nearby. A chair, at least 2 pillows and a small mat is required for each participant. Plenty of cold drinks must be available. If no music system is installed a portable cassette player can be used. Remember, batteries should be on hand in case there is no suitable source of electricity. Tapes for each type of exercise will be the personal choice of the teacher. **NB.** Anyone using recorded music for classes in a public building must ensure they are covered by a PPL (Phonographic Performance Limited) licence for the premises, otherwise they will have to purchase one for their own use. There are strict copyright regulations which govern the playing of recorded music to a group.

Clothing

Good footwear is essential to provide adequate support to the feet and help avoid strains. A loose cotton shirt may be more comfortable antenatally than a tight leotard and all women need to wear a good supporting bra.

AQUANATAL EXERCISES

Aquanatal exercises are supervised group activities for the ante or postnatal periods which take place in water. The exercise sessions are performed to music and can be executed in standing, lying, kneeling or squatting positions. It is not necessary to be able to swim to participate. There is a growing interest in these sessions and more and more women are requesting them.

Facilities

Ideally the sessions should take place in a swimming pool which is closed to the general public and where the water temperature can be increased to at least 28-30 degrees centigrade. The surrounding air temperature should be the same as that of the water to prevent chilling. Cooler water is not conducive to relaxation, but if the water is too warm, it may lead to vasodilatation, hypotension, fainting and fatigue. Hospital hydrotherapy pools will be too warm unless the temperature can be significantly reduced. An ideal depth would be to the level of the xiphisternum. If the depth of the water increases to above the level of the xiphisternum, vertical balance is threatened *(Dyson, 1990)*. However if there is insufficient depth, some movements could be performed kneeling or squatting in shallower water to allow the level to reach the optimum. Women should wear a bra in the water to support the breast tissue and should avoid jumping movements to prevent breast discomfort.

There may be a music system available which can be used as long as this is not loud enough to drown the exercise instructions! If there is no such system, a portable cassette player can be taken along, but make sure that it is a battery-operated one. For absolute safety, stand the player on a towel, away from the splash area, and ensure that hands are dry before adjusting the controls.

The women must have access to warm showers immediately after the exercise session and to a room in which they can have a warm drink. If there is no provision for the latter, women can be asked to bring a flask with them. The drink is necessary as blood sugar levels and blood pressure may drop following exercises in water. A private room would allow the participants to rest and discuss posture, lifting techniques, breathing or parentcraft topics.

Equipment

There should be at least two, preferably more, floats for use by each woman. If the swimming pool is unable to provide sufficient floats, it may be possible to purchase these from parentcraft funds as a small charge is often made for aquanatal classes. Alternatively large clean empty plastic receptacles eg. 2-litre milk containers, can be a cheap substitute.

Staffing

Adequate staffing levels are an important safety precaution. At least two professional staff and one lifeguard are needed at every session unless one professional has life-saving qualifications. The professionals may be an obstetric physiotherapist and a midwife, or, if this is not possible, two midwives may run the sessions provided one has aquanatal qualifications. In the latter case, the exercise content should be discussed with an obstetric physiotherapist beforehand. The assistant midwife will be in the water with the women to assist and correct.

Clothing

Women may wear anything comfortable e.g. maternity swimsuit, leotard or bikini with 'T' shirt over the top. It is recommended, however, that they also wear a sports bra for extra support of the breasts. The physiotherapist or midwife who is on the pool-side should wear a loose-fitting cotton 'T' shirt over a swimsuit, or possibly legging-type bottoms which will allow correct postures to be seen easily by the group. Non-slip trainer-type footwear is essential.

Benefits of Aquanatal

Water is an excellent medium for the performance of exercise. It has beneficial effects on the musculoskeletal, respiratory and cardiovascular systems. McMurray et al. (1990), found the plasma beta endorphin was significantly elevated when exercise took place in water during pregnancy. This may explain the psychological feeling of well-being of the pregnant woman following aquanatal sessions. The buoyancy of the water supports the weight of the body allowing easier movements with less strain on joints. The increased body weight and the change in the centre of gravity have much smaller effect during a non-weight-bearing exercise *(Revelli et al., 1992)*. The pressure of the water may help to reduce lower-limb oedema and stimulate bowel function and the resistance of the water around the chest wall will help to improve respiratory function. If the temperature is adequate and floats are available, water is an excellent facilitator of relaxation.

Contra-indications

The women participating in antenatal or postnatal aquanatal regimes should be carefully checked against the following criteria which could be contraindications to group therapy in water:

- heart disease
- respiratory insufficiency
- infections
- diabetes
- epilepsy

Women with the above conditions would not be included unless their problem is minor and they are monitored frequently. (This latter criterion might mean that extra members of staff would be needed).

Women with specific **pregnancy-related** conditions including the following should also be discouraged from antenatal sessions:

- history of spontaneous abortion
- shirodkar suture (cervical cerclage)
- pregnancy-induced hypertension
- ante-partum haemorrhage
- intra-uterine growth retardation
- ruptured membranes
- history of premature labour

If a problem has settled, for instance early bleeding in pregnancy, a letter from the consultant obstetrician stating that the woman is fit for aquanatal exercises would be required. If a woman presents with musculoskeletal problems, the midwife should consult with an obstetric physiotherapist before the woman joins the group.

Postnatal contraindications would be:
–   unhealed perineum
–   vaginal discharge
–   any infective condition

Again, if a woman presents with any musculoskeletal problems, the midwife should consult with an obstetric physiotherapist before the mother is included in the group.

Antenatal

Any session should always start with a general warm-up routine which may be carried out in or outside the pool. The "warm-up" serves to start to increase the load on the cardiovascular system, to mobilise the joints and to keep the body warm if the water is rather cool. This part of the routine can last up to 10 minutes.

The following input will be in the water and can include some moderate aerobic work intended to increase the heart rate and so improve cardiovascular efficiency. Care should be taken not to allow the women to exercise too strenuously as this could raise the body temperature in over-warm water and be potentially harmful for the baby (see Page 121). However, when exercising in water of 30 degrees centigrade, body heat is evenly and effectively dissipated so maternal temperature is very unlikely to exceed 37 degrees centigrade *(Rocan, 1984)*.

Fig. 11.1 Exercises in water

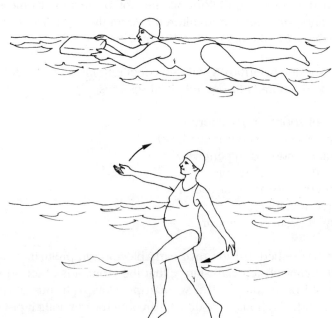

The aerobic part of the session can include:
- circulatory exercises
- pelvic tilting
- posture
- pelvic-floor exercises
- squatting
- gentle pelvic rotation
- muscle stretching - including hip adductors
- swimming

The above should not continue for more than half an hour, gradually slowing down with stretching, before a period of general relaxation in the pool using adequate floats. If the water is not as warm as recommended, it would be wiser to omit the relaxation period in the pool.

Postnatal

Diastasis must be excluded before performing any trunk rotations postnatally (see Ch. 8). Stretching need not include the hip adductors. All other exercises may be performed more quickly than in the antenatal period.

Points to remember when teaching aquanatal exercise

For any trunk movements, the level of the water must reach the xyphisternum to ensure the abdominal corset is supported by the water. It may be necessary for the women to kneel if the water is not deep enough. Even though the abdominal corset is protected by the hydrostatic force of the water, any rotation exercises should be performed with great care to avoid the possibility of diastasis of the recti (see Ch. 2).

The speed at which movements are performed in water affects the difficulty of the activity - the faster the movement, the harder the work. This knowledge can be used to progress individuals postnatally.

Care must be taken to avoid overtiring the women as they may not realise the workload they are undertaking and become fatigued. They should feel pleasantly exhilarated not exhausted.

Exercise in water must not take place directly after a meal as cramp of the extremities is more likely when digestion is taking place. If it is not possible to arrange the session for mid-morning or afternoon, advice must be given to the women to have a light carbohydrate-rich snack about an hour before the start. Toe-pointing exercises should be avoided as they often lead to cramp during pregnancy.

Safeguards for the Professionals

This is a list of points that should be agreed when planning aquanatal sessions (you may wish to add others):

- women to be at least 16 weeks gestation
- written permission from their consultant obstetrician or general practitioner
- women to be screened correctly
- no contra-indications should be present
- a comprehensive record of appropriate personal and obstetric details to be kept
- correct pool temperature to be maintained
- check safety of pool surrounds and access to emergency telephone
- pool regulations must be observed
- two professional staff and a lifeguard must be present at all times if neither professional has a lifesaving qualification.
- maximum number of 10-12 women
- the group to be strictly observed at all times
- no more than forty minutes of exercise to be performed
- fatigue, chill and overheating to be avoided
- women not to be allowed to over-exert themselves and produce pain
- avoid increased lumbar lordosis
- warm drink to be available afterwards

Midwives who would like to set up aquanatal classes in their area will need to:
- establish a local need
- investigate local venues
- contact their obstetric physiotherapist about the possibility of a joint venture for advice
- contact their midwifery manager about support, funding, cover, insurance
- discuss advertising methods
- decide on policy, screening procedures and relevant forms

The midwife should be able to swim and ideally, would hold at least the Bronze Medallion in life saving techniques.

Aquanatal sessions are beneficial during pregnancy and postnatally and encourage a healthy life style for the family where baby and family sessions are held. Above all THEY ARE FUN!

SUMMARY OF ADVICE FOR EXERCISE TEACHERS:
- to check there are no obstetric complications or pre-existing disease.
- to avoid hyperthermia, especially during the first trimester.
- to start activity slowly - warm up - build up the exercises and then cool down gradually.
- to exercise one area of the body and change to a different area for the next movement.
- to avoid positions which increase lumbar lordosis or stress on the symphysis pubis or sacroiliac joints.
- to ensure that exercises should be performed slowly and accurately.
- to ensure that those women who are not accustomed to exercise do not over-exercise initially - little and often is the ideal
- to encourage women to take time, to stretch and get up slowly after relaxing.

WOMEN SHOULD BE REMINDED TO:
- avoid exercising if feeling unwell.
- avoid vigorous exercise in hot weather.
- drink frequently whilst exercising
- avoid lying flat on the back after the fourth month of pregnancy.
- listen to your body - if you feel dizzy or very breathless, STOP AND REST.
- stop before you feel tired.
- avoid holding your breath during an exercise.
- exercise within the limit of individual comfort and ability.
- start with a few repetitions and gradually increase.
- if you feel pain - STOP.
- remember that as pregnancy advances, the level of exercise will decrease.

ALL TEACHERS OF EXERCISE-TO-MUSIC AND AQUANATAL SHOULD BE FULLY QUALIFIED TO DO SO BY ATTENDING AN APPROVED COURSE AND REACHING THE REQUIRED STANDARD OF A RECOGNISED BODY IN THESE FIELDS.

**WOMEN SHOULD ONLY BE DIRECTED TO CLASSES
RUN BY QUALIFIED PROFESSIONALS**

References

Artal R., Wiswell R.A. Eds. *Exercise in Pregnancy*. Baltimore: Williams & Wilkins. 1986.

Ashton J. Antenatal and postnatal classes with a difference. *Journal of the Association of Chartered Physiotherapists in Obstetrics and Gynaecology*. 1992;70:15

Bush A. Cardiopulmonary effects of pregnancy and labour. *Journal of the Association of Chartered Society of Physiotherapists in Obstetrics and Gynaecology*. 1992;71:3

Clapp J. The course of labour after endurance exercise during pregnancy. *Am. J. Obstet. Gynecol.* 1990;163(6):1799

Huch R., Erkkola R. Pregnancy and exercise, exercise and pregnancy: a short review. *Brit. J. Obstet. Gynaec.* 1990;97:208

Jacobson B., Smith A., Whitehead M. *The Nations Health: A strategy for the 1990's*. London: King's Fund, 1991.

McMurray R.G., Berry M.J., Katz V. The beta endorphin responses of pregnant women during aerobic exercise in the water. *Medicine & Science In Sports & Exercise*. 1990;22(3):298

Polden M., Mantle J. *Physiotherapy in Obstetrics and Gynaecology*. London: Butterworth Heinemann, 1990.

Revelli A., Durando A., Massobrio M. Exercise and pregnancy: A review of maternal and fetal effects. *Obstetrical and Gynecological Survey*. 1992;47(6):355

Rocan S. Aqua fitness - an overview. *Fitness Leader*. 1984;March 2.

Sady S.P., Carpenter M.W. Aerobic exercise during pregnancy. Special considerations. *Sports Medicine*. 1989;7(6):357

Wallace A.M., Boyer D.B., Dan A., et al. Aerobic exercise, maternal self-esteem and physical discomfort during pregnancy. *Journal of Nursing and Midwifery*. 1986;31:6:255

Wolfe L.A., Hall P., Webb K.A., Goodman L., Monga M., McGrath M. J. Prescription of aerobic exercise during pregnancy. *Sports Medicine*. 1989;8:273

Further reading

Association of Chartered Physiotherapists in Obstetrics and Gynaecology. *Guidelines for Aquanatal Classes*. 1990. (Available from ACPOG secretary, c/o CSP., 14, Bedford Row, London WC1 4ED.

Baum G. *Aquarobics*. London; Arrow Books Ltd., 1991.

Donovan G., McNamara J., Gianoli P. *Exercise Danger*. Western Australia: Wellness Australia Pty Ltd. 1988. (Available in UK from Fitness Leader Network, P.O. Box 70, Fareham, Hants. PO14 4HT.

Fletcher G. *Get Into Shape After Childbirth*. London; Ebury Press. 1991.

Whiteford B., Polden M. *The Postnatal Exercise Book*. London: Frances Lincoln, 1992.

Video tapes

BBC Pregnancy and Postnatal Exercise Video
    (Ashton J., Conley R., Polden M.)
    BBC Publications. 1991.
Y Plan Before and After Pregnancy Video
    (Gaskell J. Jennings M.) London Central YMCA. 1991.

Useful contacts

For details of training courses for teachers of exercises to music contact:
Royal Society of Arts (RSA) - Tel:0203 470033
Royal Society of Arts Examination Board,
Progress House,
Westwood Way,
Coventry, CV4 8HS.

Sports Council - Tel: 071 388 1277
16, Upper Woburn Place,
London, WC1H 0QP.

London Central YMCA - Tel: 071 580 2989
Training and Development Department,
112, Great Russell Street,
London, WC1B 3NQ.

For details of training for teachers of aquanatal exercises contact:
Aquarobics Ltd. - Tel: 081 878 9868
143, White Hart Lane,
Barnes,
London, SW13 0JP.

For details of PPL licences contact:
Phonographic Performance Ltd. - Tel: 071 437 0311
Ganton Street,
London, W1V 1LB.

Appendix

ITEM	NAME & ADDRESS
Beanbags	
Matchett Bags	Cuneiform The Old Post Office, Weasenham Road, Gt. Massingham, Norfolk, PE32 2EY.
Birth Cushion	
Gardosi birth cushion	Teasdale Hospital Equip. Stockport, SK3 0AN.
Cushion	
Valley cushion	U.T. Care Products Ltd., Unit 3, Dearne Enterprise Centre 1, Barnburgh Lane, Goldthorpe, Rotherham S63 9PG 0709 890655
Charts	
Antenatal and Postnatal	ACPOG Leaflet Secretary c/o CSP, 14, Bedford Row, London WC1R 4ED.
Be Comfortable Series	Farley's c/o Mrs M. Smith, Crookes Health Care, 1, Thane Road West, Nottingham NG2 3AA.
Childbirth Charts Growing Uterus Charts	NCT Maternity Sales Burnfield Avenue, Glasgow G46 7TL. 041 6335552

A New Life Series

Cow & Gate
Film Librarian,
PO Box 99,
Trowbridge,
Wiltshire.

Female Reproductive System
Infertility
Male Reproductive System
Pregnancy and Birth
Conditions for Caesarean Section

E & S Products Ltd.,
A2 Dominion Way,
Rustington,
W. Sussex. BN16 3HQ.
0903 773340

Childbirth Graphics

Anatomical Charts

Adam, Rouilly Ltd.,
Crown Quay Lane,
Sittingbourne,
Kent ME10 3JG.
0795 471378

Antenatal Exercise Programme
Postnatal Exercise Programme

Chartex Products
International Ltd.,
Unit 1, 20, Grasmere,
Liden, Swindon, Wilts.
SN3 6LE.

Leaflets
Guidelines for Aquanatal Classes
Care of your Body (set of 3)
Pregnancy
The Birth
Postnatal Exercises
Advice following Caesarean Delivery
Hysterectomy Advice Leaflet
Exercise & Recreational Sport
 during Pregnancy and after Childbirth
Pelvic Floor Exercises for Stress
Incontinence

ACPOG Leaflet Secretary
c/o CSP, 14 Bedford Row
London WC1R 4ED
Tel: 071 242 1941

Mats
Airex

CME
7, Ascot Park Estate,
Lenton Street,
Sandiacre, Nottingham.
NG10 5DL.
Tel: 0602 390949

Nomeq
23/24, Thornhill Road,
Redditch, Worcestershire,
B98 9ND.
Tel: 0527 64222

Dunlopillo
See above.

CME

Models
Embryological Development

Adam, Rouilly, Ltd.,
See above.

Fetal Doll

Pelvis

E.S.& P. Ltd.,
See above.

Pelvis with ligaments

Pelvic Floor

Pelvic Supports
Fembrace   - pelvic support

Tubigrip

Seton Products Ltd.,
Turbiton House,
Oldham, OL1 3HS.
Tel: 061 652 2222

Promedic - pelvic support
Trochanteric Belt

Promedics Ltd.,
Clarendon Road,
Blackburn,
Lancs. BB1 9TA.
Tel: 0254 57700

Transcutaneous Electrical Nerve Stimulators (TENS)
Promedics Obstetric

Promedics Ltd.,
Clarendon Road,
Blackburn,
Lancs. BB1 9TA.
Tel: 0254 57700

Spembly Pulsar

Spembly Medical Ltd.,
Newbury Road,
Andover,
Hants. SP10 4DR.
Tel: 0264 65741

Videos

The BBC Pregnancy and Postnatal
Exercise Video by ACPOG members

The Y Plan Before and After
Pregnancy Video by YMCA

ACPOG Book Secretary
c/o CSP
14, Bedford Row,
London WC1R 4ED.
Tel: 071 242 1941

Wrist-splints

Futura wrist-splint

Promedics Ltd.,
Clarendon Road,
Blackburn,
Lancs. BB1 9TA.
Tel: 0254 57700

Wrist-splint

Seton Products Ltd,
Turbiton House,
Oldham, OL1 3HS.
Tel: 061 652 2222

Wedges

Right angled

Harrison Bedding Co.
Westland Road,
Leeds, LS 11.
Tel: 0532 771255

Nottingham Rehab.
Ludlow Hill,
Nottingham, NG2 6HD.
Tel: 0602 452345

Relyon Ltd.
Wellington,
Somerset, TA21 8NN.

Useful Addresses

Association of Chartered Physiotherapists
in Obstetrics & Gynaecology
Tel: 071 242 1941

(ACPOG) c/o CSP
14, Bedford Row,
London WC1R 4ED

Aquarobics Ltd.
Tel: 081 878 9868

143, White Hart Lane,
Barnes,
London SW13 0JP

Health Visitors Association (HVA)
Tel: 071 378 7255

50, Southwark Street,
London SE1

National Childbirth Trust (NCT)
Tel: 081 992 6762

Alexandra House,
Oldham Terrace,
Acton, London.
W3 6NH

Royal College of Midwives (RCM)
Tel: 071 580 6523

15, Mansfield Street,
London, W1M 0BE.

Royal Society of Arts (RSA)
Tel: 0203 470033

Progress House,
Westwood Way,
Coventry, CV4 8HS.

Sports Council
Tel: 071 388 1277

16, Upper Woburn Place,
London, WC1H 0QP.

Y.M.C.A - London Central
Tel: 071 580 2989

112, Great Russell St.
London WC1B 3NQ.

Index

Posture
  normal 22-23
  in pregnancy 22-23, 34-40
  in puerperium 73, 77, 90-91

Pregnancy
  physiological changes 19-24
  physical problems 24-26

Progesterone
  effects of 19-24, 72-73

Prolapse 30, 79

Psychoprophylaxis 5, 54

Pubococcygeus 17

Puborectalis 17

Pudendal nerve 18

Puerperium
  physiological changes 72-73
  physical problems 74-79

Pulsed electromagnetic energy (PEME) 74, 75, 78

Quadratus lumborum 15

Rectus abdominis muscle 11, 13-14, 15, 23, 84, 85

Rectus sheath 11, 12, 13, 14-15. 61. 84

Refresher classes 116

Relaxation 45-51
  in labour 48, 49, 53, 54, 55-57, 61
  passive 48, 50, 57
  physiological 45-48
  postnatal 49, 92
  progressive 45
  ripple 50
  teaching 49-50

Relaxin
  effects of 21-22, 73

Respiratory system
  physiological changes 19-20, 54-55, 73, 119

Rest 25, 36-37, 48, 89, 92

Reunion classes 117

Rib flare 20, 22, 25

Rib pain 20, 25

Royal College of Midwives (RCM) 6, 136

Sacro-iliac joint 8, 22
  anatomy 8
  problems 9, 22, 22, 23

Sacrum 8

Sciatica 23

Shoulder and arm exercises 40, 106-107

Special needs 114

Sport
  in pregnancy 28, 120-121
  return to 92
  to avoid 28, 120-121

Squatting 9, 58-59, 108

Statement by CSP, HVA, RCM 6-7

Stress 42-45
  effects 43, 44
  in pregnancy 44-45
  manifestations 42-43
  positions 42-43

Stress incontinence 23, 25, 73, 78, 79
  causes 23, 78
  incidence 78
  treatment 25, 79

Stretching exercises 40, 55, 108-110

Superficial perineal muscles 16

Supine hypotensive syndrome 21, 36

Support
  tights 24, 98
  pelvic 24, 26, 75, 77

Swimming 28, 127

Notes

Notes